STOP SH*TTING YOURSELF

STOP SH*TTING YOURSELF

15 Life Lessons That Might Help You
Calm The F*ck Down

Sam Delaney

CONSTABLE

CONSTABLE
First published in Great Britain in 2025 by Constable

1 3 5 7 9 10 8 6 4 2

A CIP catalogue record for this book
is available from the British Library.

ISBN: 978-1-40872-027-1

Typeset in Minion Pro by SX Composing DTP, Rayleigh, Essex
Printed and bound in Great Britain by Clays Ltd, Elcograf S.p.A.

Papers used by Constable are from well-managed forests
and other responsible sources.

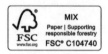

Constable
An imprint of
Little, Brown Book Group
Carmelite House
50 Victoria Embankment
London EC4Y 0DZ

The authorised representative
in the EEA is
Hachette Ireland
8 Castlecourt Centre, Dublin 15, D15 YF6A, Ireland
(email: info@hbgi.ie)

An Hachette UK Company
www.hachette.co.uk

www.littlebrown.co.uk

To Bren

Contents

Introduction

In January 2020 I became the most complained-about person on British television.

It happened on a Friday. I had been invited onto the daytime TV show *This Morning* to review the newspapers.

One of the stories they wanted me to talk about concerned some new responsibilities given to high-street pharmacists. In order to help overstretched GP surgeries, local chemists had been asked to offer more medical advice and interventions.

I decided to have some 'fun' with the story, claiming that I would personally be unwilling to accept health advice from pharmacists who were, after all, merely glorified shopkeepers.

My co-pundit, Vanessa Feltz, immediately corrected me by saying that pharmacists were in fact highly trained professionals.

I didn't doubt she was right. But the important thing for me was not accuracy – it was attention. I knew it was a daft thing to say. I was only saying it to provoke debate, to play devil's advocate, to verbalise the worst opinions of some of the dumbest people watching and – most importantly of all – to try and get a cheap laugh. I assumed that anyone watching would understand that.

I was wrong.

On social media, a few dozen pharmacists had seen the show and weren't happy with what I said. In fact, they were pretty angry. I felt as if my comments had been so self-evidently meant in jest that they were overreacting. I decided it was best not to engage with them.

But within hours there were hundreds of pharmacists expressing their displeasure about what I'd said. Someone had helpfully clipped the video of my comments and it had been shared hundreds of times. Pharmacists from all over the world waded in, some of them calling me some pretty unpleasant things, including 'awful journalist' (fair enough), 'a disgrace' (bit much) and 'a terrible father' (strange).

By that evening, I was inundated with complaints from the global pharmacist community. I had really touched a nerve. I was trending on Twitter. My email inbox and Instagram DMs were overflowing with bile and invective.

By the time I'd finished dinner, the first few death threats had landed.

My wife told me to ignore it, that it would all blow over. My kids asked me why I was so quiet and anxious. I felt silly telling them the truth: that Dad had gone on telly, made a dumb joke about the people who worked at the chemist's and now people were threatening to spike his next prescription with lethal poison.

My wife was wrong, it did not blow over. For days afterwards, I woke up to more angry messages. I felt besieged. I learned some important lessons during this period of my life, one of the most important being: do not, ever, fuck with pharmacists.

I went to ground. I came off social media and stayed indoors. I was unable to take my mind off what people were saying about me. I felt bruised, stressed, exhausted. I was disinvited from all future bookings on *This Morning*. My mind whirred for days with worry and self-admonishment.

I felt ashamed for letting it affect me so badly. I had worked in the often brutal cut-and-thrust of the British media for two decades; this was pretty bad but it wasn't my first taste of public criticism. Plus, as a mouth-for-hire who had often been paid to say or write things that were likely to upset others, I realised it was a bit rich of me to fall to pieces the moment I received a bit of blowback.

I didn't understand why I was struggling so badly. I kept telling myself I was tougher than this. I reminded myself of all the times I had survived worse situations. Eventually, I turned the anger I had initially felt towards my abusers back on myself. Why was I so fragile? I started to hate myself for feeling the way I did. I was a silly little man who went on the telly, shot his mouth off, then dissolved into a puddle of self-pity when the shit hit the fan.

I'd always tried to present myself as the sort of bloke who swaggered through life with a breezy smile, who faced down life's pitfalls and shitstorms with a cheeky wink and an adorable grin. I wanted to be accomplished, resourceful and successful in a very casual sort of way. I'd been working on this persona for the past forty years. Now, I felt as if the mask was slipping. The truth was that, despite all of my efforts to be tough and nonchalant, I was burned out, fragile and sensitive. Underneath my laddish bravado I was still shitting myself – just as I had been all my life.

Ever since I was a small boy, growing up in a raucous, single-parent household, surrounded by my older brothers, laughing along with all the mayhem, I was scared. I fixated on what other people thought about me and worried constantly about what was round the corner. I grew up in a working-class home, full of fun, love, chaos and insecurity. I think I was conditioned to be fretful from the start.

Since those days, I had cultivated a more stable, comfortable life. I had a home, a career and a family. I had worked (fairly) hard to insulate myself against the uncertainties of my childhood. But my ill-fated appearance on *This Morning* brought all of those feelings back. It showed me that, while my material circumstances might have changed, I was yet to completely heal the emotional and mental bruises I had picked up when I was a kid. I spent most of my time pretty happy and confident, yes, but it still only took a smallish knock like this to knock me back into a state of discomfort and anxiety.

'Pharmacygate' was a blessing in that it pushed me to confront all this stuff. Why, despite my life seeming to be a success, was I still scared? I had ditched drink, ditched drugs, done a bunch of therapy, got fit, fulfilled most of my professional ambitions, married my childhood sweetheart, had two beautiful kids and yet, still, I wasn't quite comfortable with myself or relaxed about the world around me. There had to be a way of life that was smoother, simpler and didn't involve a constant cycle of ambition, burnout, illness, depression and recovery.

Eventually, the *Sun* reported that my *This Morning* appearance had become the most complained-about moment of the year, with 3,496 disgruntled viewers contacting the regulator Ofcom. By the time this figure was published, Covid-19 had struck and the world was in lockdown. Suddenly, pharmacists were engaged on the frontline of the pandemic and far too busy to worry about irritating journalists making daft comments on daytime TV. Like almost everyone else, I was confined to my home, forced to take a step back from the complicated life of distraction and endeavour I had built.

The lockdown imposed an important period of reflection. As heartbreaking stories of tragedy and loss around the world mounted, I felt an overwhelming sense of good fortune. It might sound smug but it was genuinely a humbling sense of luck: a vivid awareness of my own privilege. For perhaps the first time in my life I started to feel as if I was enough. That I didn't need to keep pushing for more. I didn't need to plough every moment into the pursuit of betterment because what I had was already what I wanted.

Of course, I had to work to live, but my mindset had changed. I began to see work as a simple means to an end. I gave myself a break.

I began to read about various movements in the USA that glorified rest as an act of resistance. Many of them were political: a rebuttal to the exploitation of disenfranchised minorities by the forces of endgame capitalism. As a straight white male with a mortgage and a media career, I couldn't claim to be a disenfranchised minority. But I was nonetheless transfixed by the notion of the so-called 'soft life'. It was a movement that consciously eschewed the social, economic and cultural forces that have driven generations of human beings to exhaust themselves mentally, emotionally and spiritually. I started to reflect on how these forces had shaped my life and my sense of identity: the anxious and lustful pursuit of money that had been instilled by a combination of my insecure childhood and the turbo-consumerism that surrounded me in adulthood. The professional ambition that was informed by my low self-esteem. And the desire to be respected as a man – to be cool, to be tough, to be smart, to be funny. To be productive, to be driven, to be almost machine-like in my actions – consistent, relentless, emotionless.

Yes, despite my fantasy that I was somehow above the influence of masculine norms, I realised I was just as vulnerable to them as the next dickhead. Like so many other men of my generation, I was engaged in life as a competition. I had been indoctrinated with the idea that the world was split into winners and losers. Being a winner seemed attractive but avoiding becoming a loser was the real motivation. I had to win. This had been drummed into me by the house I grew up in – as one of four boisterous brothers – by the school playgrounds where I was educated, the terraces from which I watched football as an adolescent, the pubs I drank in through adulthood and the workplaces where my career had played out. I realised that I had been engaged in a constant battle for attention, edge, admiration and, ultimately, supremacy. I was performing at all times – as the man I thought I should be rather than the man I was. It was exhausting. No wonder it made me unhappy.

A year after my *This Morning* performance, I went on YouTube and reviewed it: a neat encapsulation of the inauthentic way I had been living. I was suited and booted, slathered in make-up, beaming from ear to ear as I spouted meaningless bollocks for cheap laughs and attention, while contriving a Jack the Lad air of cocksure indifference. But I was not indifferent, was I? I was a scared little boy who fell to pieces when people started criticising the things I had said. It was the wake-up call I needed: there was a gap between who I really was, deep down, and who I had been pretending to be. Resolving to close that gap for the sake of my sanity was one thing. Working out who I really was, deep down, felt like a much bigger challenge.

A couple of years ago I wrote a book about how and why I got sober just after turning forty. I explored the factors in my life that had been responsible for my escape into booze and drugs. The themes that kept coming up were work and masculinity. I worked too hard because I was scared of failure. And that fear was rooted in my idea of masculinity: I felt that I needed to be successful, respected and resourceful. As old fashioned as it sounds, I felt as if I needed to be a provider to my wife and kids. And like all men, I had a toxic sense of competitiveness inside of me that made me want to keep pushing everything to the limit: the amount I achieved, the amount I grafted, the amount of admiration I could attract from others.

There is something very exhausting about being a bloke. The pressure you put yourself under to pursue all these fantasies. I call them fantasies because they are not rooted in any practical reality. I don't think any of us are born wanting to be Johnny Big Bollocks. I think we pick up these mad ambitions and vanities as we go along: from our peers, our family and the deranged world of money and consumerism that surrounds us. Of course, women are just as vulnerable to this stuff and a great deal more besides. But I can't really write with any credibility about the difficult experience of being a woman. I do know that there are millions of men like me who have been artificially programmed to compete to be the best: to be strong but sensitive, fun but philosophical, an attentive

8

father but a committed professional who always works late and replies to emails at weekends. It's a lot. It can feel suffocating. It drove me to drink and drugs for a while. It drives thousands of men a year to take their own lives. I think it's time we talked about it more: the confusing, tiring and toxic business of being a modern man. On the one hand, we are told by society to 'open up' more, to talk about our feelings and be a bit more vulnerable. On the other hand, we are told that being a man is so easy.

I happen to believe that it is easier to be a man than a woman, especially a straight white man who lives in an affluent part of the world. But that doesn't mean that we should be forbidden from expressing our fears, our troubles, our insecurities and our pain. We have to stop feeling guilty about having feelings. Having feelings is part of being human.

When I came of age in the nineties, there was a beautifully simple template for masculinity. It was called 'laddism' and drew on the simple pleasures of football, hedonism and irreverence. We were the generation who took nothing seriously, especially ourselves. When *Loaded* magazine first came out it was a breath of fresh air for lads like me. Previously, glossy magazines aimed at men had told us all to aspire to strange, James Bond-type archetypes. Fast cars, expensive watches, luxury travel: it all seemed a bit elitist and alienating. But *Loaded* elevated the lifestyles of ordinary blokes to being something exciting in themselves. It didn't matter where you lived, how much money you had or what your parents did for a living: we all had it in us to go out and have a great time with our mates as long as we adopted the right attitude. And that attitude should be one of reckless nihilism. Not gonna lie, it was fun while it lasted. At the outset, *Loaded* set the tone for a refreshingly democratised form of masculinity: funny, smart and inclusive. But over the years the idea of laddishness drifted into something more tawdry – the mags that followed in *Loaded*'s path (some of which I worked for) began to focus more on cheap titillation and moronic juvenalia.

The personal fallout of that scene was pretty deep for many of the participants. If you spend years going out of your way to avoid any semblance of self-reflection and just cope with life's challenges by going down the pub, you're going to get your comeuppance at some point. I can honestly say I don't know many blokes of my generation who haven't had to face their demons in middle age one way or another. Depression, addiction, relationship woes: the chickens were bound to come home to roost. We just hadn't ever bothered to find sustainable ways of managing our emotions. Distraction was our only strategy.

Nowadays, there has been a huge shift away from that nineties brand of laddish frivolity. Social media influencers promote a new type of hyper-serious masculinity. There is Andrew Tate, the cage fighter turned crypto-bro, who tells his millions of young male acolytes that women are manipulative but stupid and that all they must care about is money and cars. Tate flaunts his personal wealth and muscular body as evidence that his cynical, serious, fascistic design for life is the only feasible route to happiness for modern males. Worryingly, millions believe him.

At the less aggressive end of the scale, there are the self-help brigade who have swamped the podosphere with advice on how to better yourself as a man. The likes of Andrew Huberman, David Goggins and Joe Rogan (and in the UK, the former sports presenter Jake Humphrey) use the language of business and science to define modern masculinity. Theirs is a world of 'high performance', 'protocol optimisation' and 'marginal gains'.

It is the lexicon of mechanical engineering applied to human beings. It feels to me as if these men are more comfortable seeing themselves as machines than as people. Machines can be rendered efficient and predictable; they can be refined and improved; crucially, they are unburdened by emotion.

I often wonder if these guys ever got over watching *Robocop* in the eighties. In case you haven't seen it, it was a movie about a man who died and was rebuilt as a metal-plated fighting machine with no heart or feelings but a massive gun and a computer for a brain. An alluring role model for an adolescent boy, maybe. But there is something sad about wanting to be that dead-eyed and emotionally numb in adulthood. It suggests a certain fear of what feelings might do to you. Yes, your heart can be the source of great pain. But it is also what brings us joy and love and wonder. These are the most important parts of being alive. They are the privileges of being human. I feel like the new gang of masculinity influencers are a bit ashamed of their own humanity. They are telling young men that to feel things is inefficient. That perfection is a legitimate goal. That all happiness lies in constant progress. It doesn't half set us all up for failure. Worst of all, it's really boring. None of those guys ever seem to be having much fun. Silliness is not something they have managed to optimise yet.

This book tells the story of how I learned to lean in to a different type of masculinity. It took me years of pain and fear and chaos to understand that all the other versions I'd tried just didn't work for me.

The experience of lockdown showed me that I didn't have to live life at a breakneck speed or push myself constantly. That rest was an end in itself. That competitiveness was futile and often toxic. That I could find happiness by just calming the fuck down.

By the way, when I talk about the importance of relaxation and the futility of hard work, please don't think of me as a foppish dilettante, lounging about on his sofa all day, writing poetry and wondering why the peasants bother working so hard. I have always had to work for a living. I grew up in home where my mum worked full time in low-paid jobs supplemented by state benefits to feed my brothers and me. And while I have enjoyed some success and a huge amount of fun in the course of my career, I've not made enough dough to protect me from financial insecurity. I work to pay a mortgage and feed my family just like millions of others. I'm not saying everyone should down tools and live off the land. We all need to work, yes. But we all need to show ourselves a bit of compassion along the way, take our foot off the gas when we can and under-stand that we are good enough, just as we are.

Neither am I saying that ambition or self-improvement is bad. The high-performance stuff is great for those who are built that way. Some people require and relish the constant setting of goals. If it makes them happy, that's great. I'm just here to say that it is possible to accept who you are right here and now. You don't have to be constantly moving forward. You are allowed to stop and smell the roses. And if someone throws a bucket of shit on your head while you do so, don't panic. You will cope.

In this book, I explore the influences that shaped the man I used to be: unsure of myself, preoccupied by gaining the acceptance of others and hungry for easy distraction. Next, I look at the price I paid for living that way: the way in which I neglected my own physical, mental and emotional health and never quite learned how to make myself happy. Part of this relates to my struggles with drink and drugs, something I wrote about in my last book but is so entwined with my sense of identity and my attitudes to work that it warrants a revisit here. And lastly, I describe the life I have learned to live in middle age and the pleasure I find in the simple, the peaceful, the humble and the everyday stuff that is readily accessible to us all.

Since I started banging on about my own struggles with all this mental health stuff I've found that other peo-ple will approach me, discreetly at first, to talk about their own 'issues'. It's never nice to hear about a friend feel-ing shit but, I'll admit, I feel good about being of service.

I used to be scared of admitting my own fragilities. Since I conquered that fear (some would say I have become way too comfortable with sharing my feelings) I have ended up advertising myself to others who might be struggling in silence. They will tell me that they are worried about their drinking or some other bad habit. Or that they are stressed out and don't know how to cope. That they feel overwhelmed, as if they are drowning in their own lives. Often, they can't quite verbalise the way they feel, much less why they feel that way. They just wake up every day feeling ... worried. Fearful. They're scared but they don't know what of. It is confusing. I am not an expert or a pro so I can't diagnose or cure. But I do know how they feel because I have been there myself, lots of times. I try to listen and demonstrate understanding. By doing so, I hope to make them understand that these feelings are normal. They are not alone and needn't feel ashamed because I – and millions of others – have gone through similar periods of bewildering, unspecified pain, anxiety or sadness. This is why 'sharing' gets talked about. There is a point to it: it helps others trapped in a state of sadness and shame understand that what they are going through is, while fucking horrible, a normal part of the human condition. Others have been through the same and come out the other side. There is hope.

A couple of years back an old mate who was having a wobble with his mental health got in touch. We went for a walk and he tried to explain what he had been going through. There were a few money worries, work worries, parenting worries and relationship worries. None of them were gigantic or unusual, he admitted. Just the daily shit so many of us have to deal with. The little bits of worry and pressure that slowly build up and start to weigh you down. But whereas he'd always been able to muddle through this stuff in the past, he suddenly felt like he couldn't cope. His mind buzzed constantly with worst-case scenarios and catastrophic speculation. He was struggling to sleep. He felt tense at all times. And all the usual stuff that helped, like music or exercise and just hanging out with mates and talking bollocks, just wasn't working. 'I don't think I'm depressed,' he said. 'But I'm not happy. I don't know what I am.'

'I know the feeling,' I said. 'It's like you're constantly shitting yourself about something or other.'

'EXACTLY!' he replied, with the mild excitement of someone who suddenly felt seen. 'I'm shitting myself. I can't stop. Why am I constantly shitting myself?'

I was chuffed to have successfully diagnosed his condition. But I wasn't able to offer him a simple remedy. My prognosis was positive, however: he would start to feel better eventually. Time helps. Perspective too. But probably the biggest thing is acknowledgement. Men often refuse to acknowledge their own fear, especially if there doesn't seem to be an obvious and 'legitimate' source. Unless we are being shot at or chased by a wild animal, we are unwilling to admit that we are scared. It's conditioned from the playground. 'Are you shitting yourself? Why are you shitting yourself? Look at him, everyone! He's shitting it!' These are the sort of phrases that most of who grew up male in the late twentieth century have used to antagonise others and have had used against us too. Shitting yourself is a Boy Sin. It is shameful. It is weak.

But of course, it isn't. If you want to be really tough, you could start by showing a willingness to admit to fear. And not just fear of big scary monsters. Just the low-level fear generated by the slings and arrows of everyday life: the bills, the frustrations, the daily commute, the lack of sleep, the pressures and expectations that we put on ourselves. The non-stop niggles about our health, our career, our relationship. The endless news cycle that pumps fear and dread into our weary minds. No wonder we're shitting it. I've called this book *Stop Shitting Yourself* because I wanted to put something on the cover that might catch the attention of the ordinary bloke who is a bit sceptical about wellness and self-care and feelings and that. The sort of bloke who has, like me, grown up being conditioned to suck it up, demonstrate strength and never sweat the small stuff. The sort of bloke, who despite his best efforts to be strong, sometimes shits himself all the same because, well, life can sometimes just feel like an avalanche of tiny disappointments and frustrations that is enough to crush you some days.

I want blokes like that to pick up this book and laugh because I have used not one, but two swear words on the cover and thus understand that I am not the usual sandal-wearing, bullshit-spouting mental-health guru or big- watch-wearing, ice-bath-bothering, high performance grifter. I am just a bloke who has felt the strain of everyday life and, on occasion, allowed it to drag him under. And who, in the process of getting better, learned a few things about how to cope and stay positive. Spoiler alert: it all starts with looking after yourself and doing less. It's about lowering your performance, not striving to push it higher. It's about calming the fuck down.

I hope that in reading about my transformation from goal chasing, hyper-ambitious, knackered, pissed-up dickhead to enthusiastic advocate of the soft life, you might be tempted to try it out for yourself. Just a little bit, maybe. I can't promise that it will make you rich or get you a six-pack. But you will have more fun and probably manage to calm down a bit. What more do you want?

Chapter 1

Stop Shitting Yourself About Fitting In

The day before my son started secondary school, I felt an urge to offer him a bit of advice: I just didn't know what that advice should be.

I had enjoyed a reasonable school career, with an OK social life and passable exam results. I hadn't died. I wanted him to experience, at the very least, something similar. But how had I managed to navigate myself through those tricky times? I couldn't recall. I felt as if I had stumbled through it all, mostly. There had been no real strategy or plan. I had managed to keep my head down whenever it felt prudent to do so, open my mouth when I thought it might help and hide in toilet cubicles when things got really hairy.

I'd had a few mates around me, which helped. Not because we were all kind and supportive towards one another. Quite the opposite: we were absolute fucking arseholes to each other. Back at school, you're twice as vicious towards your closest pals as you are to your worst enemies. But having mates at least meant I was able to have a laugh; I was able to distract myself from the general grimness of school life by mucking about endlessly with boys just as idiotic as I was. And by having them around me, I was able to avoid feeling lonely. Fear of loneliness is not something a young lad would want to ever admit to. But it was very real and very raw inside of me and, I suspect, most of my peers. Being alone at that vulnerable age can feel scary.

The night before he started Big School, I really had to fight the urge to tell my son this: 'Try to fit in. Nothing matters as much as fitting in, son. Look at how everyone else is acting and try to act the same way. Literally, mimic the other boys. Laugh at their jokes. Go along with their bullshit antics, even when you know deep down they are stupid or a bit mean. Shit, you should even think about neglecting your learning if it helps the other lads accept you. You'll have plenty of time to be yourself in adulthood. For now, just fit in.'

I had fallen over myself to fit in at school. The trouble was, I got so good at fitting in that, by the time I left, I had forgotten who I really was. I had become an amalgam of all the different personalities I had contrived to gain acceptance. Fitting in is a nasty habit that eventually swallows you whole.

I had been bullied for a couple of weeks at infant school. Every day at playtime, two older kids waited for me by the playground entrance. The larger of the two would grab me by the collar and pull me into a corner, then instruct me to stand facing the wall for the whole of playtime. If I turned around, he said he would thump me. So I did what he said. His pal just giggled and snarked while the big lad muttered abuse in my ear for twenty minutes. It was quite an effective bullying technique because it was low-key and undramatic. He was bullying in plain sight. He never actually had to hit me because I always obeyed his orders. Any onlookers would have just thought the three of us were playing a quiet and peaceful, if slightly strange, little game. But I can vividly recall the lump that swelled in my throat, the tears that stung my eyes and the boulder that filled my stomach every day when playtime approached and I knew I'd have to be their prisoner once again.

One day, it all got too much and I just burst into tears.

A dinner lady, who was also a friend of our family, asked what the matter was. I caved in and told her what had been going on. She collared the offenders and sat us all down on a bench to conduct an investigation. Once she'd established that the bigger lad was the instigator she looked him in the eyes earnestly and said, 'You know Sam has three older brothers in big school? Shall I tell them to come over here tomorrow and beat you up?'

He gawped back at her. I think I was as shocked as he was. I had figured she was just going to send him to the head's office. But this was a straightforward threat of violence: this dinner lady didn't fuck about.

The bully remained silent.

'Well?' asked the dinner lady after a moment. 'Haven't you got anything to say for yourself?'

The bully's little accomplice seemed to be loving the sheer awkwardness of the situation. 'The cat's got his tongue, miss!' He giggled. She turned on him: 'I don't know what you're laughing about, they'll beat you up too!' she said. His smile dropped immediately.

(By the way, this whole exchange was a brilliant example of the power of suggestion. My brothers were bigger than these bullies, yes, but they were hardly the sort of violent goons-for-hire the dinner lady was implying. As serial truants and committed soft-drug abusers, I think she would have been hard pressed to locate them, let alone rally them to commit the sort of playground retribution she was suggesting. But that didn't matter; she had planted the seeds of fear inside the tiny brains of these bullies – and they were shit scared.)

In the end, the bigger boy cried and promised to leave me alone. His mate, obviously, fell into line. And they never bothered me again.

I got to thinking that I should surround myself with a bit of back-up. This is how I found the Donald brothers: a couple of lads from the local estate who were well respected for both their football skills and fighting prowess. My mum knew theirs, which went a long way back then, and they allowed me to hang about with them.

The younger of the two, Tyrone, once persuaded me to do a runner out of school in the middle of the day. I was no rebel. I was too nervy, sensitive and guilt-prone to do anything as cool as run away from school in broad daylight. Or so I thought: Tyrone's charisma was hypnotic. The fact that he had chosen me as his accomplice in this audacious scheme was so flattering. He was respected in the playground, on the estate and beyond. He had marked me out as a worthy accomplice. How could I refuse him? And so one day, during morning play, he grabbed my arm, gave me the nod and together we sprinted for the gates, out of the school and all the way up the street towards the shops. There we were spotted by the school caretaker, Mr Leeds, exiting the newsagents. 'Oi! What are you two up to?!' he shouted. We lost our bottle, pulled a U-turn and ran straight back into school. Hardly the stuff of Ronnie Biggs, but a respectable escape bid for a couple of eight-year-olds.

We got in trouble for that and I – not for the last time – burst into tears while confessing my crimes to my mother that evening. Characteristically, she brushed it off and told me to learn from it. She thought my mistake had been to follow my cheeky, boyish instinct for misadventure. But she was wrong: I didn't have a cheeky, boyish instinct for misadventure. I was, at heart, a coward. I could never be bothered with what seemed like the unnecessary hassle of wanton rebelliousness. I would have liked a quiet life. But my Achilles heel was, and would be for many more years to come, a desire to be liked and to fit in. That abortive attempt to do a bunk with Tyrone Donald should have been a learning experience. I should have held on to those feelings of fear, shame and remorse that consumed me when we were caught. I should have remembered the terrible sense that I had let my mum down and used the memory to steer me away from future misdemeanours. But I didn't. Time and time again I would let my appetite for affirmation and acceptance trump almost every better instinct I had.

When you're a lad there is a sense of real threat from other kids around you. Unencumbered by the civilised norms of adulthood, kids will do and say mean things pretty casually. I witnessed rough and tumble at school and in the area I lived. The best form of protection was being part of a group. I was lucky to have older brothers around me. But sometimes I thought to myself: *Who is protecting them?*

One night, when he was about sixteen, my brother Dom and a couple of his mates were chased through a subway by a bunch of drunken yobs. It was a random, unprovoked attack – the likes of which seemed quite common back in the early eighties. One of his mates, Siam, was six foot three and sported a mohawk with spikes that added another four or five inches to his height. My brother and his other pal, Darren, had shaved heads and wore Dr Marten boots. Maybe their appearance was what made them targets for random violence. As they ran through the subway, Siam fell behind. My brother turned back to help him but the assailants had beaten him to a pulp then smashed a full bottle of whisky over his head. Siam was rushed to hospital where he stayed, in a coma, for the next few weeks. When he finally came round the doctors said he had to avoid all drugs and alcohol for the rest of his life to preserve his damaged brain. But shortly afterwards, Siam took acid, jumped out the window of his tenth floor flat and died. I was about eight when all of this happened. Siam had been around our house all the time when I was growing up. The fact that he had been beaten up, almost died, then killed himself in such dramatic circumstances soon afterwards was crazy, extraordinary, terrifying and tragic. But the way I heard grown-ups discussing it made me feel as if that sort of thing was pretty normal in the adult world. That I lived in a world where those arbitrary acts of violence and death were commonplace.

It wasn't completely isolated either: there was a bloke who lived near us called Ross who was a bit of a local celebrity. Ross drove a sports car. He was funny and handsome and charming. Everyone knew him. He was always so nice to me and the other local kids. One day I heard my mum casually tell our neighbour that he had been banged up for beating the shit out of a bloke in a pub. It was discussed in a very matter of fact way, as if nobody was surprised that he had committed such an act. I remember thinking to myself: *If even nice blokes like Ross are going round beating people up, then none of us are safe!*

Then there was the lad in my year at school who, a couple of years after we left, got mugged and beaten unconscious by a gang late at night who then threw him off a bridge into the river. He was found dead a couple of days later on the banks of the Thames. At the funeral, practically everyone I knew from school turned up. We were all still young, many of us (including me) completely unsure of how to recognise, let alone express, our emotions. It was the stuff of nightmares – the kind of thing you told yourself couldn't ever really happen to someone you knew. Again, it strengthened this sense I had in the back of my mind that the world was a violent, dangerous place. That life was deeply unsafe.

My mum had a mate called Betty, who was also a single parent. She used to come over for a cup of tea and bring her two sons to play with me. They were a nice family. Eventually Betty met a bloke and got re-married. My mum went to their wedding. On their holiday, Betty and her husband died when the ferry they were travelling to Belgium on sank. We heard about the Zebrugge disaster on the news and my mum wept just at the thought of what the victims must have gone through. A day later she received a phone call from a friend telling her that Betty had been one of them.

The following year my mum attended another old friend's wedding. Two days later, she and her new husband died when the plane that was taking them to their honeymoon in New York blew up over the Scottish town of Lockerbie.

Two famous tragedies in one year. Two good friends of my mum's, both of them dead. My young mind registered my mum's grieving but filed away the idea of mass-scale tragedies that made the news and affected your life directly as just another everyday pitfall of adult life.

All of these horrible incidents, when written down together over the space of a few short paragraphs, might make us sound like the unluckiest family in the world. Or at least discourage you from ever becoming pals with the Delaneys in case the death curse might befall you next. And, yes, I suppose it is unusual – maybe a little uncanny – for one ordinary family to know so many people who died in such unusual and sudden circumstances. But the point I am making is not about the why or how these deaths happened (which I don't understand and choose not to look for any meaning in) but the way in which it shaped my emotional responses to the world at a young age. While my brother, my mum and I all mourned the loss of our friends, they also came to feel normal. I learned not to 'overreact' to tragedies. I understood death and violence to be no big deal. Or at least I learned to act as if they were no big deal. Inside, I found all of this stuff completely traumatising. But on the outside, I cultivated a veneer of resilience. This gap between how I felt and how I acted would become a big problem for me as I got older. It would take me decades to realise that it was the source of so many of my mental health problems.

* * *

It wasn't just the fear of violence; there was also the chance that other boys could make you feel small, stupid, left out or lonely. Being dragged into the corner of the playground, away from your mates, and forced to stand facing the wall every playtime can really make an impact. You worry that you will lose your mates because you're not playing with them any more. They will forget about you or, worse, resent your absence. You also wonder why no one is coming to save you: how can I, a harmless and helpless little lad, be left at the mercy of these bullies in full view of the playground? It's terrifying.

When I was ten, a new kid joined our class. He was from Egypt (a place I can honestly say I had previously assumed to be mythical) and he had the best name I had ever heard in my life: Rami Elshibiny Mohammed Elshibiny. Sensational. Rami was a good bloke with a gigantic smile, a brilliant sense of humour and a massive helmet of black curly hair. I was impressed enough to offer him playground friendship immediately.

After a couple of weeks of knocking about at school, he invited me round to his house. His mum answered the front door and pointed me in the direction of Rami's bedroom. I walked in to find him lying frontways on the bed, reading a comic while 'The Heat Is On' by Glenn Frey blared out from his portable stereo.

It was like a scene from a John Hughes teen movie, only starring a tubby little Egyptian boy rather than Matthew Broderick. I must admit, it looked rather choreographed but I respected it all the same. Before I had a chance to say 'Hi', his little brother – Basil – scuttled into the room and pressed STOP on the stereo, bringing an abrupt stop to Glenn Frey's muscular pop-rock anthem.

'BASIL YOU DICK!' blurted Rami. 'I had that lined up especially for when Sam got here!' There was a short silence before it dawned on him that he'd actually said this out loud, at which point his face flushed with shame and he stared down at the floor.

I didn't say anything because I knew exactly how he felt. He had worked overtime to impress a new mate and it had all gone wrong. He was exposed as a person who gave a shit about what other people thought about him. This was a mortal sin for young lads of our (or, to be honest, any) age. Basil laughed and ran out of the room. Rami and I stood in awkward silence for a while, then endeavoured to move past the whole embarrassing incident by playing with his Action Force figures.

A few weeks later, I witnessed a playground scuffle. Rami was being attacked by another kid in our year, Carl. I was surprised that this was happening because Rami was personable as fuck and Carl was not usually the violent type. Instinctively, I thought I'd better stick up for the new kid. I ran over and punched Carl on the nose, causing blood to erupt from his nostrils. I was quite pleased with myself at the time – but this was not the first or last time I discovered that the fleeting thrill of violence was swiftly followed by a deep sense of remorse and shame. I reckon I must have punched about six people in the face in my life, the majority of them before the age of thirteen. Each time it left me bereft, as if I was acting against my nature. Sometimes other lads would cheer me on and I would feign pride. But inside I was crying, wondering what my mum would make of it all or just telling myself I was a cunt.

A few years back I found out via Facebook that Carl had died suddenly. It made me feel guilty all over again for punching him unnecessarily back in 1985. I was much bigger than him. I confessed my remorse to my mate Ollie who tried to make me feel better by saying: 'You can only beat what's put in front of you, Sam.'

* * *

Of all the recreational drugs I have ever tried, my least favourite is marijuana. And yet, strangely, it's the one I've consumed more than any other. I remember going back to a mate's house after school, aged fourteen, to try my first spliff. There were four of us – we'd all chipped in to purchase a fiver's worth of hash, facilitated by someone's older brother. One of us rolled a truly appalling joint and we passed it round. I had never even smoked a fag so didn't know how to inhale. I remember I couldn't stop talking due to my nerves. After my first puff, I just carried on jabbering bollocks to my pals, the smoke billowing out of my gob as I did so. My pal Ben, the oldest and tallest of the group (a boy who had extraordinarily lavish stubble from an early age, which basically made him our de facto leader) admonished me sternly for 'wasting money' by failing to inhale.

The next time I tried, I managed to suck some smoke into my lungs and thus experience the sensual impact, which I disliked greatly. It made me feel uncomfortable, nervy and nauseous. But everyone else seemed to be having fun so I said nothing and took another toke. That was in 1989. I carried on with this ludicrous masquerade for another twenty-six years. Smoking dope (we called it 'puff') was so ingrained in my culture that I genuinely didn't feel as if I had a choice. In adolescence, I wasn't someone who bought it, but that was mainly because I couldn't afford to. I used to get a fiver a week pocket money from my mum, and an eighth of weed cost fifteen quid. I could never work out how all my pals managed to buy such large amounts.

I went to a comprehensive school in a pretty middle-class area and there were a lot of kids with rich parents who had more money than me. They often funded their own habits by selling and buying bulk amounts in deals financed (knowingly or not) by their parents.

I remember getting laughed at once for trying to convince a mate to go halves with me on £7.50's worth of weed (a 'teenth'). Everyone else was putting together deals to buy ounces of the stuff and I was scrabbling about purchasing about two spliffs' worth for £3.25. That followed me around for a few years after ('Remember when Sam tried to go halves on a teenth?'), and the piss taking was fair enough. But the weird thing is how humiliated I felt for being unable to buy larger amounts of a drug I actively disliked. Being a teenage boy is fucking stupid.

Even when I got to university and made a few new friends I found myself weirdly drawn towards those who liked to sit around smoking and getting high. By this stage I had at least lost my sense of constant financial insecurity. I was the first in my family to get to university and I qualified for a government grant (yes, they still gave those out back then) because I was from a low-income household. My dad – who lived in a separate household which was not low income – offered to pay my rent. It was the first time in my life I felt somewhat financially stable. I found myself smoking all day and night for much of my university career, growing perversely accustomed to the accompanying state of anxiety, lethargy and paranoia. It was all done to assimilate. Maybe if I'd fallen in with a bunch of, say, sci-fi fanatics at school, I would have gone on to seek out similar tribes at university and beyond. I might have been happier and healthier as a result. But I fell in with a crowd who liked sitting about all day with bloodshot eyes, watching *Neighbours* and forgetting their own names. Not that getting high defined everyone's personality. The truth is that most of my mates liked music, mucking about, having fun and making each other laugh. Those are the sort of people I've always liked to hang around with. I guess people who are fun, creative and not overly bothered about rules are more likely to be the sort of people who like to get high. So there was a logic to it. Don't get me wrong, I always liked the idea of getting high. I just didn't like the reality of it very much. It not only made me feel sick, it was often fucking boring too. I don't doubt that my mates were genuinely having a great time. We all react to different substances in different ways. When I got older and discovered cocaine, I absolutely loved the feeling it gave me for the first few years, while there were pals of mine who found the sensation unbearable. They were shrewd enough to simply not take coke because why would they take something that they didn't enjoy? I was not so logical in my lifestyle choices. I carried on puffing that sickly stuff despite all the horrible things it gave me, including panic attacks, seizures and – on a few occasions – episodes of public incontinence. I think that I reached a stage where I didn't really notice that I didn't like it. It was just normalised, like drinking water or breathing air. It wasn't really a case of whether I liked it or not – it was just something I did. Weird.

It was a symptom of the chasm between my true self and the person I projected to the world. The gap between these two identities sometimes made me feel like shit. But the thing about lads is that we don't want to seem like we care about anything. To be 'manly' is to be indifferent. What is it that makes that sort of man – the type who never flinches, never shirks and rarely smiles – so appealing as a role model? Maybe it's because they appear to be unencumbered by human emotion. Emotions are unpredictable, messy and often unmanageable. They make us think, feel and behave in irrational ways. They represent our 'variables'. They undermine our ability to control situations. Sometimes it seems as if we'd all be better off without them. What appeals to many blokes is the ice-cold heartlessness of the sharp-shooter, who is able to navigate life with precision, control and unerring logic.

But it's just not realistic to try and live like that. Life is unpredictable and chaotic. You can't control everything. That can feel scary. I spent years kidding myself that control was possible. To numb my fear of an arbitrary universe, I burned myself out with work and worry, while managing the side-effects with booze and drugs.

I listened to a podcast interview with Paul Weller, one of my all-time heroes. The interviewer asked him if he thought he was a genius. 'I don't,' said Paul. 'I just think I'm really good at being me.' That's something I think we should all aspire to. But to be really good at being yourself, you must have the courage not to fit in. When everyone in his school was a punk, Weller decided to take inspiration from the mods who had been fashionable over a decade beforehand. When everyone else wanted to listen to loud, thrashing, angry music, Weller listened to soul. When the other kids wore torn T-shirts and leather jackets, he wore suits and ties. And he continued to buck trends throughout his career: when all his fans wanted more of The Jam, he disbanded them and started a new group that played pop-jazz and wore boating blazers. None of this was a self-conscious bid to be different. It was simply his willingness to do what he liked. To wear what he liked, listen to what he liked, say what he liked. To be himself consistently, unapologetically and defiantly. In a world that often cajoles us into alien roles designed to appease others, getting good at being yourself takes real bravery. That's what makes it so rare and it's why simply leaning into your own values, your true identity and your better instincts is enough to make you stand out from the crowd. But fuck me, it's tough. I am not a genius. But unlike Paul Weller, I've never been good at being myself either. Although I have been getting better at it recently.

I grew up in a small street where the neighbours included a builder, a salesman, a domestic cleaner, several unemployed people, a sewage worker and a burglar. In my house, there was a secretary (my mum), a milkman (my mum's boyfriend) and a postman (my brother Dom).

I understood that their jobs, their appearance and their social status were not reflections of their intelligence, humanity or value as people. I loved some of them, respected most of them, liked the majority and tolerated the milkman.

My brother Dom pounded the streets of Central London, delivering mail in the rain after leaving school at sixteen. He hated it but it earned him money that allowed him to chip in to the housekeeping. My brother Cas left school a year after him (also aged sixteen) and became a benefit-claiming, stay-at-home stoner for a year or so. Dom resented Cas's slovenly lifestyle and used to verbally lay into him every night when he got in from work. Until one night, Cas could take no more and smashed his dinner plate over Dom's head, mid rant. A potato flew upwards and stuck to the ceiling. We didn't own a step ladder so, somehow, the potato remained up there for several months. It was a chilling reminder of the ugliness of fraternal violence.

Anyway, years later, Dom and Cas ran a successful production company together. There was no plate smashing or weed smoking by then. They were driven, smart and ambitious. Like my other brother, Theo, who didn't live with us back in the plate-smashing days, they were inspirations to me.

Our parents split up when we were kids and we were left to grow up in pretty difficult circumstances, cared for by our mum while our dad disappeared up the class ladder with a new career, a new family and a big new home on the other side of town. Did that sense of rejection make us determined to prove ourselves as worthy? Did the financial insecurity of our childhood make us fearful of poverty and driven to succeed? Did the heroism, hard work and incessant positivity of our mother – who raised us with unswerving love and kindness and good humour – give us the confidence and resolve we needed to succeed? I think so, yes.

I wouldn't want my kids to grow up in exactly the same circumstances as I did. But I do think that a certain amount of adversity gives you the resilience and determination that can help you thrive. More importantly, I think it can stop you from becoming entitled or arrogant.

My sense of identity, my sense of self-worth, my self-esteem, my confidence, are all rooted in my background. I lived my childhood in social housing surrounded by love and anxiety. There was never much money, there was always insecurity but it was all offset by a sense of fun and emotional warmth. In the eighties, council housing started to get a bad name. The government was selling off council homes; private ownership was everything. Living in a place that belonged to the local authority was looked down on. This stuff has an effect on your sense of identity, however hard you try to fight it.

Council estates, like any other parts of our communities, contain all sorts of different lives and fascinating stories – some good, some bad. I spent my whole childhood in social housing and have no grandiose conclusions to make beyond the fact that there was never any central heating so it got fucking cold in winter.

The media likes to report on social housing in a binary way: the people who live there are either dangerous dole-scroungers or heroic families triumphing against the odds. The only constant is that to grow up in council accommodation is to be dealt a bad hand that you will struggle to recover from for the rest of your life.

Most of us pay someone or other for the right to live in our home: whether it's the bank, a private landlord, a local authority or a housing trust. Council houses come in all shapes and sizes. My mum still pays rent to the council to live in the house I spent most of my childhood in. I own a home (or at least my bank does, until I pay them off in about twenty years) that used to belong to the council. On the street where I live, half of my neighbours are council tenants. Some of the people I went to school with now live in social housing; some live under the yolk of intimidating mortgage repayments; I know of one or two who were lucky enough to have homes basically bought for them by rich parents. Comprehensive schools, like council estates, comprise an array of human life that might seem surprising to some who've never stepped foot in either.

When I was in my early forties I found myself working as a radio host on a national news and current affairs station. One evening I was invited by the company to join the senior execs at a special dinner with members of the Conservative government. As one of the only left-leaning presenters at the station, I was surprised that I was the sole host to be invited – but felt pretty certain that their first five or six choices just weren't available. Anyway, this dinner was held inside the company's headquarters, with private caterers serving gourmet grub in the boardroom. There were half a dozen high-profile politicians in attendance. I had interviewed most of them in the past – one in particular (who subsequently rose to one of the very top jobs) I'd gotten a bit pally with. I've never been much of a fan of Tories, but this fella seemed down to earth enough: chatty, not too posh and up for a laugh. He greeted me warmly and I could see my corporate bosses were impressed.

I felt as if I was behind enemy lines but, at the same time, was pretty pleased with myself for being there. I found myself at ease among these powerful folk and able to speak with them comfortably, in spite of the fact I disliked their politics. *So this is what it's like to be a grown-up*, I thought to myself. I was happy to be socially adaptable.

Yes, I had grown up in a working-class environment. But my dad, after he'd built his new life of money and success elsewhere, had exposed me to middle-class stuff, like nice restaurants and the occasional foreign holiday. I understood that this was a privilege that enabled me to fit in with a diverse range of people. Yes, I thought to myself, an evening with a bunch of public schoolboys who run the country is a walk in the park for me. They aren't to know I'd have them up against the wall once the revolution finally gets going.

But as the evening wore on, the fine food was gobbled up and the expensive wine guzzled, things got weirder. The point of the dinner was not explicit but it soon became apparent that this was an off-the-record forum for frank and unapologetic exchange of views about the relationship between the media (us), politicians (them) and society (everyone else). There was a great deal of robust BBC bashing. There were some decidedly off-colour gags about poor people being chucked around. One of the politicians made an unkind comment about council house 'dwellers'. Another spoke about the return of grammar schools. I had clammed up because (a) I was the only sober person there (b) I had no idea what role I was supposed to play in this peculiar soirée and (c) I was scared they might at any moment bash me over the head and start feasting on my dead body.

But I thought I had better contribute something so I piped up about grammar schools, asking the group, 'But what happens to the kids who don't pass their eleven-plus?'

'They get sent off to a comprehensive with the other thickos,' replied one of the gang, through a mouthful of beef.

'I went to a comprehensive!' I replied.

'Well, that makes sense!' said someone else. And they all roared with the laughter of privately educated men with bellyfuls of free food and booze.

Was I ashamed, humiliated or upset? Not really. I laughed along with them. There are worse things you can call me than thick. But it was a reminder of the way in which we can be casually judged on the basis of superficialities and stereotypes.

It has often happened to me the other way round. A bloke I know at West Ham complained to me once, 'You're an all right bloke but you're a bit...fancy, aren't you?'

'In what way?' I asked.

'Well, all those long words and that. You just sound quite posh.'

Strangely, this hurt me just as much as being labelled a thicko by a Cabinet member. ''Scuse me for having read a few fucking books!' I protested.

The point is, people will judge you for perceived differences wherever you go. I'm not complaining because I am lucky to have lived a life that has allowed me to traverse different social environments with relative ease. But that shit bothers you along the way. People will always try to find reasons to get one up on you. Sometimes, they make the most of the fact that they are richer, stronger, more successful. Other times, they'll do the opposite and insist that they've had it so much harder than you. You can either pander to this bullshit by adjusting your personality to blend in with any company you happen to find yourself in, performing constant social contortions to render yourself safe from criticism. Or you can just lean in to being you. The second option is much harder because it requires you to know and like who you are. This is something that would take me many years to work out.

Chapter 2

Stop Shitting Yourself
About Money

Insecurity about money is something most of us grow up around. If we are lucky enough to get our hands on some when we grow up, we guard it jealously and fret non-stop about the possibility of it disappearing.

Due to all the shame and confusion so many people feel about class and where they 'fit' into society's hierarchies, they cling to their financial status as the key arbiter of success. If you don't have a fancy background, didn't get much of an education or you do a job that isn't necessarily regarded as having much inherent kudos, you will always emphasise your ability to earn as the only true marker of success. Which is fair enough. Money is nice and to earn it feels good. But often people – men especially – use money as a club with which to beat down others. In the ongoing micro-battle for superiority that exists between all blokes, money is the most commonly used weapon. And I'm not saying I've only ever been on the receiving end: throughout my life, whenever I've been lucky enough to be flush with cash, I have flashed it about. This is partly down to the chip on my shoulder: I want all those snobs and Tories to know that they're no better than me because, look, I've managed to make just as much as them despite their head start.

I have been self-indulgent and performative with my dough. I have acted cool about it too, as if money means nothing to me beyond the access it allows to pleasure and comfort. But I am not in the least bit relaxed about money. I'm fucking terrified of the stuff.

Throughout my life, through good times and bad, money has been a constant source of anxiety. Being skint is miserable, of course. But even when I've had plenty in the bank, I've never been able to shake the low hum of stress that accompanies any thoughts of finance. If I haven't got much, I worry incessantly about where the next pay cheque will come from. If I've got a few quid in my pocket, I stress about how to organise it, spend it and manage it. I worry about losing it through naivety, irresponsibility or frivolity. I am just not comfortable around money.

I appreciate that I am luckier than many: I own my home and I can put food on the table. But money worries aren't always rational. We live in a society that is obsessed with money and links it closely to status and self-worth. We all know deep down that our bank balance is not an accurate reflection of our value as human beings, but sometimes it's hard to remember that. Our financial situation can shape our sense of personal success and failure. It can conjure feelings of shame and inadequacy. It can sometimes feel impossible to shake these feelings, however irrational you know them to be.

When I was a kid, my mum was always skint and would talk about it constantly. The house was strewn with lists of incomings and outgoings, usually scribbled manically on the back of envelopes containing final demand letters. She was a single parent surviving on a part-time secretary's salary plus the government's family allowance payments. I'm not saying we were poverty stricken – we always had food to eat – but money was the source of constant anxiety. From an early age I imbibed the idea that personal finance was a perilous and terrifying aspect of adult life. But at least my mum was happy to admit her problems and discuss them with her mates, many of whom were in a similar boat.

Middle-class life is different: people can be guarded about their money worries. They want to appear relaxed, comfy and perhaps a little smug. It's like a conspiracy of silence, wherein nobody admits that they're skint and so we all end up thinking we're the only one.

It's almost impossible to switch off from this stuff. When I wake up in the morning, I get a text from the bank telling me about the state of my overdraft. Then I get a notification alerting me to a couple of payments due to leave my account later in the day. Next, I receive an email from the credit rating agency I foolishly subscribed to, telling me that my rating has just dropped from 'good' to 'fair' for reasons they are unable (or unwilling) to explain. And all this before I finish my first cup of tea.

A therapist once warned me, 'It's all too easy to bury your head in the sand about your financial problems.' I wish that was the case. I wouldn't mind five minutes' respite.

When you meet posh people, irrespective of how much money they earn, they seem so relaxed and blasé about their finances. There is an assumption through good times and bad that they will find a way through. It annoys me that there are people like that. It shouldn't, but it does. I resent people who are careful, shrewd and orderly in their financial affairs. Because, personally, I am only ever one late invoice payment or surprise gas bill away from an emotional meltdown.

As a self-employed person, I have become accustomed (but by no means comfortable with) a feast-or-famine mentality. I have rarely saved, have spent irresponsibly at times but have generally lived a good life. Certainly, I've enjoyed more stability than my mum did when I was younger. As a result, I am reluctant to moan about money or admit to suffering from financial anxiety. I am haunted by an inner voice that says that I have no right to fret about money when there are millions of people living with far greater problems than me.

But financial worries, at whatever level, are a huge source of mental illness. If you feel like you can only speak out about your worries if you are in a state of acute poverty then you keep them inside and – just like any secret problem – they mutate into feelings of shame and isolation. Studies show money worries are one of the biggest factors that encourage people to consider suicide. People are more likely to turn to drink and drugs to cope with financial stress. Mental health issues make it harder to earn, and so the cycle continues.

In certain social circles, saying 'I'm skint' can provoke pretty awkward responses. I find it quite entertaining, in a way. Some people just can't get their heads around your willingness to admit that you're short of a few quid at the end of the month. But I consider myself to be doing societal service. As with any problem, it's always worse when you think you're alone. Once your trouble is out in the open and you start to realise there are a ton of other, perfectly decent, people going through the same sort of thing as you, you feel so much better. You are less ashamed, less lonely and less likely to descend further into dark and destructive thought patterns. Even better, you have the support and acceptance of other people like you.

So when people ask how I am, sometimes I will tell them casually, 'I'm a bit skint at the moment to be honest, it's shit.' For me, it is cathartic. For them, it might be a helpful reminder that they are not alone.

* * *

An addictive personality can manifest itself in numerous ways. Since I quit booze and drugs in 2015 I have channelled my obsessive tendencies through an array of other outlets.

To begin with, it was work. I spent the first three years of sobriety distracting myself from the feelings that still lurked inside by taking on as many jobs and money-making schemes as possible. For as long as it all kept delivering me cash and (superficial) kudos, I was satisfied. I had yet to realise that I wasn't really addressing the feelings and hang-ups that had caused me to drink for so many years. I was just coping in a different, slightly less destructive way.

For a few years, I felt pretty rich. Not Elon Musk rich. Not even Mike Baldwin rich. Just rich by my own standards, which meant I never had to worry about bills or mortgage payments and could afford to take my family on holiday a couple of times a year.

It was at this time that I discovered another compulsive behaviour common among recovering alcoholics: spending. I got into the habit of buying stuff online to make myself feel happy, important, successful or excited. Most of all I think I did it to stop myself from feeling bored. I was terrified of boredom and had spent the previous three decades trying to avoid it by getting shitfaced. Now that was off the agenda, I turned to my credit card for help.

I would buy things to elicit the little hits of dopamine that lager and cocaine had once delivered. The money that used to go to the local publicans and dealers was now being diverted to overpriced clothes shops and electrical gadgetry stores that caught my eye on a Sunday-morning scroll through Instagram.

My wife started to comment on the stream of boxes that were being delivered daily, containing more trainers and jackets than I had time to wear. I told her it was fine, we could afford it. I told myself I deserved it. But this pattern of self-indulgence as a form of 'reward' was as familiar as it was destructive. It was a mutated form of the same old addiction: a futile hunt for validation, distraction and tiny, fleeting thrills.

The whole time I was spending to numb the bad thoughts, I was deferring the real work of unpicking painful feelings. To understand where they came from, reflect on their toxic impact and try to find some closure. To try and be a better person who was more comfortable in his own skin. The sort of person who could find enough comfort and pleasure in his life without needing those constant, empty, short-term hits of synthetic joy.

I ran into some business problems in 2018 that made me knock the spending on the head for a while. It also left me with a bit of extra time on my hands. Sometimes, the universe intervenes – forcing you to change and take care of yourself a bit better. I had to slow down, reflect and focus on the recovery work I had been avoiding for the previous three years of sobriety. That meant therapy, groups, rest, fitness and time spent with the right friends and loved ones.

I came out on the other side far from perfect but immeasurably happier in myself. I learned to cope with the insecurity, shame, anger, pain and anxiety that had always been part of me. I worked hard to understand where it all came from. That helped me to move on from it. I no longer needed to crush my feelings with booze, drugs, work or spending. I could sit with my feelings and watch them pass.

I've been back on my feet for five years now – with my work, money, health, sobriety and emotions far more stable than they have ever been. Instead of trying to tell myself and others that I was OK, I chose to face up to the fact that I wasn't. I faced my demons. I stopped buying as many trainers and I began taking naps in the day. Not every day, just the ones that feel a bit overwhelming. Most mornings I walk my dog in the park without headphones so I can hear the birds singing, then I come home, put a record on and make a pot of tea.

Chapter 3

Stop Shitting Yourself
About Being a Man

I don't know if you've ever been punched in the face while driving on a dual carriageway at 60 m.p.h. but I have and, I can tell you, it's not pleasant.

It was late one night in the early noughties and I was driving some pals home from a football match. One of them, someone I was very close to, sat next to me in the passenger seat, pissed off his nut (having tried to drink off the pain of yet another West Ham defeat on a cold and rainy night at Upton Park).

We had somehow managed to get into an argument about the American invasion of Iraq. Something I said angered him and, from his position in the passenger seat beside me, he managed to land a left hook on my nose, just as I was descending the flyover heading west on the A13. I swerved across a couple of mercifully empty lanes before regaining control of the car, pulling over and instructing him to get the fuck out.

I'll never forget his parting shot as he exited the vehicle. He booted the door and shouted, 'Fuck you, I don't want a lift in your shitty car anyway!'

How. Fucking. Dare. He.

I mean, disagree with me over US foreign policy, fine. Punch me in the face, sure. But call my car shitty? That really overstepped the mark.

Some context: the car was a five-year-old Peugeot 306 which I had purchased from my girlfriend's mum a year previously at a heavily discounted price. It wasn't exactly flash but it was the best car I'd ever owned at that stage of my life. Before that, I'd only driven proper old rust buckets, the type you bought for a few hundred quid and which broke down every five minutes. The Peugeot had a CD player and working air con. To twenty-six-year-old me, it felt grown up and classy.

When he wasn't drunkenly attacking me, this mate of mine was someone I usually admired and respected. He was a decade older than me and, like a lot of the older blokes I hung around with, he'd worked his way up from humble beginnings to make a big success of himself. I can't remember what car he owned at the time but it would definitely have been a very expensive one.

This is why his remark about my motor stung so badly. I can honestly say that the next day, when I woke up with a bruised nose, it was the words 'shitty car' that echoed round my mind more than the violence. I felt hurt at the suggestion that I was small time and pathetic, that he was too good for my crappy hatchback. That I was unsuccessful, unglamorous, maybe even unmanly.

This was the level of insecurity I carried around with me at that age. I think a lot of young men feel the same. Masculinity is something we learn to express in pretty limited ways: often it's through the things we possess. Cars are one of the big statements we can make about ourselves: we feel like they reflect our taste and sophistication but also our success and our wealth. These are the things that feed our egos.

I wanted respect from this older, richer, more successful man. It tore me apart to think he looked down on me.

I was a young man consumed and controlled by an extremely fragile ego. I was unable to forge my own criteria for what 'success' was; instead, it was handed to me by other blokes who were just as insecure as I was. I was too afraid to stop and reflect on what I felt about who I was. I just wanted other people to admire and possibly envy me.

These were all clues to the struggles with drink and drugs I had ahead of me. I was insecure, unsure of who I wanted to be, uncomfortable with a lot of my feelings and constantly trying to distract myself with external comforts. Work, money and ambition were, as it turned out, interchangeable with booze and drugs.

Don't worry: I haven't become a Buddhist, much less a communist. I like nice things. I enjoy earning and spending money. I've been skint and I've been flush and I know that flush feels much nicer. I think the notion of being careful with money is a boring means of preventing ordinary folk from enjoying themselves. I find posh people who are careful, awkward and understated about their money to be unbearably smug and dreary.

All that said, I realise now that there is a difference between enjoying the comfort and convenience that money can offer and linking your own value as a human being to your bank balance.

As it happens, that bloke who punched me is still my friend. Neither of us drink any more. He hasn't punched me in years! And I can't recall ever falling out again over geopolitics either. When he got sober, a few years before me, I saw his ego slowly deflate in a way that was quite beautiful. He was still funny and smart. But he no longer worked so hard to prove his credentials with corny displays of wealth, success or physical violence. He became vulnerable and I admired him for it. And, eventually, I wanted to try it for myself.

This male desire for status, wealth and respect among young men is even more rampant today than it was back when I was getting punched in the face on the A13. While our dads and grandads grew up with a sense of assurance around career and their role as domestic breadwinner and authority figure, things today are a lot less certain. Family set-ups are different. Rightly, men cannot feel quite so entitled to positions of dominance. The neat post-war life trajectory of education, apprenticeship, career ladder and retirement has been eroded by the forces of globalism, technology and endgame capitalism. Women are pretty angry about the raw deal they've experienced for the past few thousand years. There is resentment in the air and the words 'toxic' and 'masculinity' have become permanently entwined. I can see why this has happened and am not here to make a case for the reclamation of men's rights. For fuck's sake, lads, grow up and stop whinging about the fact that the game is up for arse-grabbers and unequal pay.

That said, this new landscape has provided fertile ground for a new brand of masculinity, grounded in rage and self-pity.

If young blokes grow up being told that they are toxic just by virtue of their gender and are grouped with all the very worst mansplainers, gropers, abusers, exploiters, perverts, dickheads and sleazy Hollywood executives of this world, then their self-esteem will suffer. When a grifter like Tate, with a six-pack and a fleet of Bugattis, slides into their YouTube feed and tells them that they don't have to feel guilty and that, in fact, they should lean into their most base and objectionable instincts, then obviously they're going to find that appealing. If he doubles down by saying that it's actually women – with all of their unreasonable demands and opinions – who are the real baddies, then you can see why a nerdy and vulnerable adolescent lad, consumed by frustration and insecurity, might be inclined to get behind Tate's moronic philosophy. Like any cult leader, Tate prays on the vulnerable. Some people suggest that we need more positive male role models to combat the appeal of Tate and his ilk.

While I'm all for positive role models, I have come to believe that masculinity is just a silly notion contrived by stupid movies, crass advertising people and idiotic chancers like Tate.

My criteria for what makes someone worth hanging around with – whether they are a man, a woman or anything in between – are based on how fun they are, how kind they are and how generous they are. Intelligence is a bonus but not an essential (some of the thickest people I know are also the kindest and most fun, so, go figure).

There are no inherently masculine traits. Some blokes are mean and moody, some blokes are kind and silly. Neither is more archetypal than the other.

Sometimes people tell me that it is 'instinctive' for a man to want to be a 'provider'. That's not true. Some men want to provide for their families. Numerous others abandon their responsibilities for an easy life. Some just want a quiet, simple life without any dependents. Similarly, there are just as many (if not more) women who have a strong instinct to provide for and protect their families. Some people step up in life, some people don't: gender has nothing to do with it.

There's a lot said about how it's important for men to feel strong while also allowing themselves to be vulnerable. To share their feelings while maintaining their core masculinity. Why? We're not kids who need someone to tell us we're tough in order to feel better about ourselves. It's the equivalent of a woman saying that she wants to be regarded as, say, a strong and decisive business-person while also being reassured about her fragrant femininity.

When I think of the word 'masculinity', I think of seventies medallion men with tight jeans and hairy chests, pinching women's arses. It's corny and embarrassing. It seems weak and insecure to require approval on the basis of your strength or emotional indifference or willingness to doggedly make advances on disinterested women. I mean, go out on the pull by all means, lads. Slap a bit of cologne on and unbutton your shirt if that's your thing. But don't make out that we all have to do it to be a real bloke.

And by the way, I am not entirely guiltless. I spent most of my younger years drinking beer, misbehaving at football and chucking about casual sexism in everyday conversation as if it were all just knockabout fun. I still fart, burp, spend too much time watching football and often shout too loudly in pubs (albeit while sipping a zero per cent beer). I spent the late nineties and early noughties working on lads' mags. I am not advocating for the abolition of the beautifully stupid tropes of the twenty-first-century lad. It's fun to be a bit of an idiot sometimes. But it doesn't make me more of 'a man.' That's not really the point. There's no such thing as a real man. There is such a thing as a real human. We are all different, all flawed, all struggling to get along but all capable of love and kindness. Accept yourself for who you are: a Muscle Mary with a fast car, a sensitive poet with a bicycle, a beer-guzzling geezer on the last night bus home or a heady mishmash of all this and more.

Being a man is not a choice between one extreme or the other. Being a man is just like being a woman. The rules are always the same: be kind, be fun, be generous, try not to take yourself too seriously. Just don't be a dick.

Chapter 4

Stop Shitting Yourself About Mental Health

I was eight years old when I got snowed in at my auntie's cottage in Gloucestershire. I had gone to visit my cousins and was supposed to be staying for one night. Even one night away from home was a big deal to me at that age. I would miss my mum, feel anxious and get tearful quite easily. I was not a very chilled kid, to be honest.

When I came downstairs after a fretful night of sleep in my aunt's cottage I was alarmed by what I saw outside. Deep, white snow as far as the eye could see. My aunt's place was nestled inside a picturesque Cotswolds valley. The snow rolled on and on across fields and up hillsides. It was like the whole world had been encased in sugar. It might have been one of the most beautiful things I'd ever seen but I was only focused on the deep sense of foreboding that had crash-landed in the pit of my stomach.

'Isn't it exciting?!' My auntie beamed. 'We're snowed in! What an adventure! We won't be able to leave the house for days! It will be just like camping!'

I did not think this news was exciting. I was not in the mood for adventure. And even at the age of eight I already knew I fucking hated camping. My infant mind was thrown into a state of mild trauma. It was horrible. I had to fight back the tears and paint on a smile to reassure my auntie that I was OK.

It's funny the way we spend so much time when we're kids trying to reassure adults. You'd think it would work the other way round. But I remember constantly putting on elaborate performances to convince grown-ups that I was perfectly OK even when I wasn't. I'm not sure where that shit comes from. Maybe I just thought it would break my auntie's heart if she knew how absolutely fucking desperate I was go home.

I called my mum at work to tell her I wouldn't be able to come home until the snow thawed in a few days. My auntie and cousins sat around watching me. I tried desperately to sound happy on the phone. But my mum knew me well enough to know that the situation would have sent me into a tailspin.

'Are you sure you're all right, Sam?'

'Sure!' I said through a manic grin, my eyes beginning to sting as I fought to hold it together. 'It's exciting! In fact, it's just like campiiiiiiiiiiiiiiinnnnnnnnnnnnnngg.'

With that, my voice cracked, then ascended into a high-pitched wail. Tears followed, with the snot bubbles close behind. Reader, I had fucking lost the plot over a bit of snow.

I know exactly what I sounded like because, to this day, my auntie still does a fucking funny impression of the episode. She was kind but I discovered, years later, that she had low-key found the whole thing absolutely hilarious. I suppose it was. But I was absolutely distraught. Why? I'm still not sure. Did I think we would run out of food and die there? Maybe. Was I really that desperate to swap my auntie's cosy country cottage for my tiny, freezing council house on the side of the A4? Seems unlikely.

I think I was generally anxious as a kid because there wasn't a whole lot of stability in my life. My dad had left, our house was a bananas menagerie of local waifs, strays, drunks and yobs. My mum tried her best to keep things on a level but it wasn't easy with four boys to raise and only the Family Allowance to do it on. She'd have occasional boyfriends who would make cameo appearances then disappear as mysteriously as they had arrived. To eight-year-old me it all seemed chaotic and unsettling. I think I became conditioned to believe that life was inherently unstable and a bit dangerous. When anything unforeseen occurred I was quick to assume the worst. I probably thought that by the time the snow thawed and I got back to

London my family would have disappeared, there would have new people living at home, someone would be dead or I'd have a horrible new dad.

Homesickness is not something that's easy to admit to. The term alone sounds so babyish and pathetic. It's not a proper grown-up mental disorder like PTSD, is it? Post Traumatic Stress Disorder is what SAS veterans suffer from after seeing stuff that can never be unseen in brutal jungle conflicts. Homesickness is what a skittish child gets when it unexpectedly snows during a trip to the Cotswolds. It feels embarrassing to talk about it.

I still got homesick when I was a teenager. I would go away on lads' trips (sorry, but that was what we called holidays with friends in the nineties) to party resorts on the continent and spend all day moping about in my hotel room, wishing I was back home eating beans on toast and watching *EastEnders*. I would feel anxious and unhappy 70 per cent of the time, my discomfort compounded by the need to conceal melancholy beneath an exhausting 'Oi, oi, saveloy!' Brits-on-tour charade. The only respite came at night-time when I would go down the disco and drink away the bad feelings until dawn. It's really not that complicated to work out why I developed an alcohol problem later in life.

Even when I got older, the homesickness lingered. When I was twenty-six I was living with my girlfriend in Notting Hill. I had my own weekly show on national TV (OK, it was Channel 5, but still). A magazine hired me to go on a road trip from LA to Las Vegas with Chris

Moyles and his BBC Radio 1 show. All I had to do was go there, get pissed, interview Moyles a bit, write it up and then fly back to present my TV show on the Saturday. For a twenty-six-year-old journalist things couldn't have been going much better.

I must admit, the week in California was a great laugh at times. While we were in LA I got to interview John Lydon on Venice Beach. We even went to a party at the Playboy Mansion. We drove in convoy across the Nevada desert, Moyles in a vintage Jag, me behind in a people carrier, all the way to Vegas where we partied some more between bleary-eyed radio shows (actually, I never even bothered turning up for the show because I was too jet-lagged and hungover).

I mean, fuck me, what a week. I am quite aware that I sound like an entitled, moaning prick to have anything negative to say about an experience like that. But half the point of this book is to speak about shameful stuff so that people reading it might be able to relate and feel less alone (the other half is just to make myself feel better). I accept that a lot of you will nevertheless be thinking, *Nope, sorry, can't relate, check your privilege, you fucking baby*. And that's fair.

But the truth is that, despite everything seeming so cool and exciting, I was consumed by an unspecified anxiety and desire to go home. I was worried and panicked – but very skilled at pretending to be the opposite. Again, alcohol provided the only relief. As soon as I felt the anxiety start to rise up inside, I hit the booze hard. After all, that was half the point I was there.

You can see the pattern. I felt insecure, scared and uncomfortable when I was out of my comfort zone. I was overwhelmed by circumstances that I felt I really should have been able to handle. This made me feel ashamed. Hiding that made me tired and even more anxious. Alcohol was the quick and easy way to dispel everything. Drink was a cure-all – the only safety blanket I needed. And over time I became entirely dependent on it to navigate my way through life, especially when things got a bit fast-paced and exciting.

It's ironic that I tried to build my career around the pursuit of unfamiliar and adventurous experiences which I was so unable to cope with emotionally that I had to use alcohol to get through them.

Now I am forty-nine. I still like the odd bit of excitement but the desire has lessened over time. I've tried many of the things that film and TV tell you are sensational and discovered that 75 per cent of them aren't nearly what they're cracked up to be (the Playboy Mansion included).

I have been sober for almost ten years. Now I can, at last, handle being out of my comfort zone. I have spent enough time sorting out my inner demons, working out where my insecurities came from and developing skills to combat them without booze or drugs. Plus, I have a wife and two kids that represent everything that matters in my life. I can be on the other side of the world, all alone or surrounded by strangers and have inner peace. Because I know they are there waiting for me when I get home. I know they're not going anywhere. I know my life has love at the centre of it and all the other stuff that happens on the fringes is just transient. Sometimes it's fun, sometimes it's shit but none of it really matters. Life is an adventure. You could almost say it's just like camping.

In 2023, I took the family to Portugal for seven days.

The coach driver who took us from the airport to the hotel was called Eduardo. Big Dire Straits fan. I sat up front and he kept making me feel the hairs on his arm each time his favourite tracks came on the stereo. '"Sultans of Swing"! What a song, my friend! Quick! Feel my arm! The hairs, they rise, yes?'

This is all while he's speeding along, one-handed, at 90 k.p.h.

Eduardo also told me he was a member of the Algarve's top motorbike gang (he tossed me his wallet while he drove and invited me to search for his membership card, in case I didn't believe him). At one point, he took a detour to show me where he lived. There were about thirty other tourists sat up the back wondering what the fuck was going on!

I asked him how long he had lived in the Algarve.

'My whole life,' he said. 'It used to be a quiet place until Cliff Richard and Bonnie Tyler bought houses here. Then the whole world wanted to come!'

Yep, it was some journey.

Then we got to the hotel. A beautiful place. It was all-inclusive; from the moment we arrived we could switch off completely: all the meals were taken care of, so was the cleaning. Our only task was to find a shady spot by the pool, read a book and take the occasional snooze. Switching my body off was easy. Switching my brain off was trickier. The constant distractions of normal life might be toxic but, like any drug, they can become quite comforting too.

I left my phone in the room all day to avoid the temptation of scrolling social media or checking emails. All very well, but in those dead moments where I wasn't engrossed in my book, kipping or playing in the pool with the lads (i.e., my wife and two kids), my brain sat there expectantly, like a confused dog with an empty bowl at dinner time. 'Where's all the usual shit that keeps us busy?' my brain asked me. 'You know, the phone calls and tweets and transfer rumours and work stuff and all of that bollocks? Feed me some stimulation for fuck's sake, I'm bored shitless!'

But I had to be firm. I wanted my brain to get used to doing nothing. I left it, like people leave their crying babies in the cot at night in the hope they will learn to 'self-soothe'.

That's what I want my brain to do. To self-soothe like a crying baby. To learn that life can't be about constant gratification. That sometimes you just have to be happy to exist. To let the troubling thoughts and difficult feelings just drift on like clouds in the sky.

I've been in the process of training my brain like this for the past decade. But holidays are like boot camp for the idle mind. For a whole week you strip the brain naked, take a deep breath and ride out the hours and days of beautiful emptiness. I mean, if you can't be content with sunshine, lazing about and eating fancy foreign grub then when can you be? What's the point in numbing the feelings with booze? That's like running to Mummy for your bot-bot. You've got to grow out of that shit.

When I was a younger man, I did have to run for my bot-bot all the time because I just wasn't at ease with myself. I was unable to cope with the raw feelings that bubbled up on holiday. I felt discombobulated by being abroad with nothing familiar to silence the little anxieties and insecurities that were always whispering at the back of my mind. Sitting on a beach doing nothing all day didn't relax me – it just left me more vulnerable to the feelings of fear and loneliness that I was ordinarily able to ignore.

I would long for six o'clock to come around so I could start getting stuck into the booze, which seemed like the only reliable way of shutting my feelings out. I certainly wouldn't tell anyone about the way I was feeling because, well, I was on holiday. I felt I had no right to be anything other than constantly delighted and upbeat. I was able to put a pretty good front on. But by evening I was absolutely gasping for a piña colada.

The booze would get me through the evening and the next morning the darkness would come back even stronger.

This routine started when I was a teenager but even by my thirties, when the kids were little, I still had a habit of getting hammered to manage unfamiliar holiday moods. During our first all-inclusive break in 2013, I remember blithely polishing off a bottle of rosé every lunchtime. My wife gave me worried looks. I was very defensive, telling her it was what the locals did, I was on my holidays and, anyway, the fact that we'd already paid upfront meant that I was effectively 'making money' the more wine I drank.

I was a bananas pisshead, obviously. But I was still trying to convince myself otherwise. So I pretended that alcohol was integral to relaxation. In fact, it was always the opposite. Booze made me more anxious and miserable in the long run; it drained me of the energy and enthusiasm to engage properly with my family, blinded me to the natural delight that the holiday was providing and, ultimately, it left me stuck in a state of emotional immaturity, where the only way I could manage my moods was through the use of alcohol.

I got through my week in Portugal really well, I think. I'm not saying it didn't feel weird. It's always hard to adjust to the abrupt change in schedules and rhythms that holidays impose. But I've got much better at embracing it all.

Mind you, I did pick up some sort of bug at the end of the week. I went to the local medical centre where they gave me pills that sent my temperature sky high. I googled the medicine's name and it turned out it had been banned in the US, UK and most of Europe since the seventies.

The Portuguese are certainly a very laid-back people. I feel I have a great deal to learn from them.

When I was a kid, my sadness would often turn into very intense worry. It seemed to work like this: I would wake up feeling sad but not know why. My brain would start looking around for reasons. I didn't understand that sometimes there doesn't need to be a reason. Feelings don't always make sense. They are illogical. They can just visit us out of the blue. It's like catching a cold. But my brain would insist that there must be some logical reason for the way I felt and, eventually, it would just start making things up for me to worry about.

I remember lying awake one night when I was about twelve, telling myself scary stories in my brain about how all the people I loved would get sick or die. About how I would never have any friends and would grow up to be lonely and miserable. About how life was just one long, boring drag that would never get better. Where did all these pointless thoughts come from? It was just my brain playing tricks on me.

But the feelings got so bad that I started to sweat and could feel my heart pounding in my chest. My thoughts were spinning out of control and I was breathing very quickly. I now know this was my first real panic attack. I got out of bed, took my blanket into the hallway and slept on the floor outside my mum's room, just so I knew she was close by if I started dying. I know, pretty weird right? But I just couldn't understand what was happening to me. Sadness had turned to anxiety which had turned to panic and fear. It was scary and confusing.

I wish I had known how to cope with those thoughts and feelings back then. I wish I had challenged them and told myself that they were all a load of barmy, make-believe nonsense that my brain was inventing to scare me. I wish I could have identified the anxiety I was feeling. But I didn't even know what anxiety was.

I didn't want anyone worrying and I didn't want anyone thinking I was weird. So I just buried my thoughts and hid my feelings. But that only left them lurking, ready to rise up every once in a while and torment me again. It wasn't until I was a middle-aged man that I understood what those thoughts and feelings were, where they came from and how to deal with them.

Growing up in my family, one of the worst things you could say about someone was that they were insecure. My old man would use the word pejoratively about anyone who displeased him: a colleague disagreed with him at work? 'He's a deeply insecure man.' A kid bullied me at school: 'Don't worry about it, he is obviously insecure.' A pundit on *Match of the Day* irritated him? 'Look at his face! You can see how insecure he is!'

I would nod and shrug and try to imply that I under-stood how pathetic and pitiful the legions of insecure people that surrounded us really were. But I didn't understand. By which I mean, I literally didn't understand what the word 'insecure' meant. All I knew was that it was a very bad thing to be. And that I wasn't it. I knew this because my dad would tell me: 'Insecure people behave stupidly and are annoying. Luckily, you are not insecure.'

Years later I found out what 'insecure' meant. And then I realised that my dad had been wrong because, in fact, insecure was exactly what I was. In fact, I had been so insecure that I was unable to ask my dad what the word meant. I thought he would judge me for it. I only had a weekend relationship with my dad and I put myself under a certain amount of pressure to make a good impression in the brief windows of time we spent together. He seemed particularly focused on intelligence and confidence in a child. I tried my best to feign both, always feeling as if I fell short. Hence all the insecurity.

I was insecure about the way I looked, the way I spoke, the things I was interested in, the way I dressed, the way I walked; I was insecure about the very essence of my being. What was the point of me? I didn't know. I felt insecure about that. But having learned that insecurity was the deepest of all character flaws, I felt ashamed of it too. I sometimes went over the top in acting like a person who was profoundly secure in themselves. I thought that behaving with forthright assurance was the only way of making anyone like me. Often, I discovered, it had the exact opposite effect.

I'm not blaming my dad. He probably thought that by telling me I was a secure person then it would be so. It was flawed logic but probably driven by good intentions.

The truth is, everyone is a bit insecure, aren't they? To not be insecure is to have total, unwavering (and slightly weird) self-confidence. A person devoid of all insecurity must never lose any sleep over the things they have said or done or the way they are perceived by others. In fact, other people's opinions are probably a complete irrelevance to them. You might suppose that someone whose self-assurance is that watertight could lack a little empathy. I mean, if you really don't give a second thought to the way your behaviour impacts on others then, yes, you must feel wonderfully free. But I'm pretty sure it also puts you somewhere on the psychopathic spectrum. Say what you like about Charles Manson, I bet he wasn't insecure.

To be insecure is to be human. To me, a certain amount of insecurity denotes a willingness to self-reflect. Which is not only healthy for you but those around you too. If you are able to carry yourself without an iota of self-doubt then, I suppose, you must have established your worldview and convictions in childhood and not had any reason to revise them since. Which would be really impressive – but I just don't buy it.

Who on earth can charge into life without stopping to worry about the wisdom of their actions, the suitability of their behaviour, the strength of their emotional responses, the shape of their nose, the choreography of their dance moves, the style of their kissing or the length of their trousers?

Of course, you need to keep this shit under control. You can't spend your whole life fretting over every last thought and deed or second-guessing how others might react to you. You need to overcome a certain amount of insecurity or at least learn to live with it. You might not ever be 100 per cent sure of yourself but you can at least learn to say, 'Fuck it, who cares?' once in a while.

I think I've managed to get the balance right, although it's taken me the best part of fifty years. I'm able to walk the dog on a hot evening in my pyjama bottoms and a pair of flip-flops without giving a fuck what passers-by might think of me. But I still have a little voice in my head that sometimes tells me I might be imperfect, incorrect, disgusting or twattish. Who would I be without that voice? Probably the sort of boring bastard that thinks he's got life sussed.

When my company collapsed and I lost both my TV and radio shows within a month of each other back in 2018, I didn't know how I would react. All bets were off.

I remember having to cut short a family holiday in the Isle of Wight and travel back to my offices in London to inform the staff that we were running out of money and might not be able to pay them that month. They were all brilliant, talented and loyal people who had grafted hard to help me grow the business in good faith. But understandably, they all soon left and I was alone in a giant, cavernous, lonely office – the office that had been alive with creativity and industry for the past three years – surrounded by bills and my own crushing sense of fear and failure.

I was miserable, exhausted and scared of the future. I had been sober for three years and, despite the prevailing chaos, I wasn't once tempted to throw myself off the wagon. I figured that, however bad things seemed, they would be a great deal worse with a hangover. Mind you, this was the first big test I had faced since I quit drinking.

In my past life I would have undoubtedly turned to the bottle. How else might I escape the daily stresses that haunted me? My wife was very supportive but there was only so much I wanted to unload on her. I was already on prescription meds and I went to the doctor, who upped my dosage. I wasn't sure that was going to fix everything. I was already in therapy but didn't know if I could afford it any more. I felt like I needed something else. Something that didn't rely on someone or something to heal me. Something I could do on my own.

What else did people do to sort their heads out when numbing the senses with drugs and alcohol were off the table? Meditation? Yoga? These things work a treat for millions but, to be honest, I just wasn't into them at that stage of my life. I was frantic, strung out. I couldn't sleep. I felt pretty lost and alone at times.

Then I did something that was pretty alien to me. I started to own up to the fact that I was struggling. I went to a meeting of the local Andy's Man Club, a charity that runs support groups to improve male mental health. It helped. I started chatting to mates about what I was going through and the things I was worried about. I was stunned by their empathy.

Next, I started writing about this sort of stuff. A couple of articles in the newspaper about my own little struggles:

the drinking, the anxiety, the childhood stuff I'd never quite shaken off. I'd been writing for years but never with much honesty about myself. I like making people laugh and found it was easy to use humour as a means of distracting from self-reflection.

Discovering sincerity was life-changing. Writing stuff down about my own vulnerabilities, resisting the constant urge to dress it up in jokes and irony, took quite a lot of determination for a professional dickhead like me. But the responses I got from strangers and friends alike were pretty powerful. It wasn't the praise (although obviously, I loved that) but the sense that my own admissions – about insecurity, low self-esteem, worry, fear, depression – seemed to chime with others. I felt a connection, often with people who, like me, had never been able to open up about this side of themselves before. I felt less alone in my feelings and therefore less ashamed of them. I started to realise that there were tons of blokes like me who had seemingly happy, comfortable lives but nevertheless wrestled with self-doubt and sadness on a regular basis. They'd heard all the stuff about mental health and the importance of sharing but they just didn't know how to do it – or with whom.

It's all about language and tone, I think. Whether you're reading Plato or listening to a self-help podcast, the means by which we might navigate the human condition remain the same. It's just the way in which it is discussed that varies. We need as many different conversations going on about this stuff as possible so we can maximise the number of people who engage.

Blokes like me have felt left out of this conversation for a while. The fact that suicide remains the biggest killer of men under the age of fifty in this country is probably connected.

Discovering sincerity was what got me through 2018 and has seen me build a better life since, in which I am able to cope with good times and bad by being open-hearted and honest. I started a mental health newsletter and podcast to keep those conversations going and I wrote my last book, *Sort Your Head Out*, which people seemed to like. Whenever I published a book in the past I would have publicly mocked it in order to show how self-effacing I was about the whole thing. But I can't do that any more. I can just tell you that I am immensely proud of it. Sharing my truth and dropping the bullshit is better therapy than a pint of Kronenbourg and a large whisky chaser ever was, I can tell you.

As a bloke who grew up in the nineties, when drunken irony was the only acceptable means of communication, it was fucking hard to take the first step towards speaking honestly about the way I felt. But if you are struggling and feeling 'sincerity curious' I can promise you that the first step is easily the hardest. Once you get a taste of how people respond – not with the mockery and ridicule you assume but with real love and kindness that helps forge meaningful connection – you will not be able to stop. I don't ever intend to. Sue me.

When I started trying to get my head straight, one of the biggest obstacles I had to overcome was the language surrounding mental health. It was strange, cryptic and clinical and often put me off engaging with the (very useful) ideas it referred to.

Set boundaries. Learn to be your authentic self. Speak your truth.

Fundamentally, it's all good advice. But what the fuck does any of it mean? Let's be honest, those sound like bullshit terms made up by Instagram scam-artists to baffle us into thinking they're saying something more complicated than they are. The people peddling this stuff mean well. Their advice is sound. But it doesn't quite make sense. So, in case you're not immersed in the lexicon of wellness, I'll decode it for you:

'Setting boundaries' translates as 'stop letting people take the piss'. They will always take the piss, unless you tell them very clearly that it's absolutely not on. And we're not just talking about massive piss-takers who come round your house and nick the silverware, either. Even perfectly nice people take the piss without realising, with their micro-demands or passive aggressive behaviour. It's the little bits of energy and time people steal from you every day.

It's easy to become a people-pleaser, who agrees to every last favour asked of them or attends every single social event they are ever invited to. But that shit is exhausting and, over time, will wear you down. You can lose sight of your own needs amid your constant efforts to help others to fulfil theirs. Bollocks to that. Prioritise yourself. Have your own schedule and stick to it. Set some non-negotiables with your friends, family and colleagues. You don't take calls or messages after 7 p.m. Wednesday night is badminton night. And, no, you can't come to those leaving drinks for the geezer in IT support. Why? There doesn't need to be a why. Stop explaining yourself. Do what you have to do.

Now, let's talk about being your 'authentic self'. We used to call this 'keeping it real'. It means dropping the bullshit and bravado you use to protect yourself from the judgement of others.

We all have slightly different personas to fit in depending on context: I always had a work Sam, a football Sam, a family Sam and a ton of other Sams I could juggle from one moment to the next. When I was a kid, I had completely different versions of myself for weekdays with my mum and weekends with my dad. It was confusing.

As Richard Ashcroft once confessed: 'I'm a million different people from one day to the next.' I know how he must have felt. It's fucking exhausting.

Being authentic is about getting to grips who you really are, what your values are, what you want to do with your life and what really matters. You probably already know all this stuff. But it's easy to sometimes lose yourself and adopt bullshit facades to ease certain situations. Let me tell you, there is nothing more liberating than understanding your authentic self and being totally unapologetic for it, no matter what the context.

I was on a train on the way to Seville to watch a football match last spring. It was full of drunken, lairy fellow West Ham fans. I approached a seat facing a right couple of pissed-up herberts. At the last minute, I turned on my heels because I decided I couldn't face sitting with them for the next three hours.

'Oi!' they said, a bit aggressively. 'Why don't you wanna sit with us?'

I turned back, smiling, and said, 'Nothing personal, lads, but you're on the piss and I don't drink so I just wanna have a kip on my own.'

They thought about this for a moment then asked, 'Why don't you drink?'

'Because I was a massive pisshead and coke-nut so I had to knock it all on the head a few years back.'

They were delighted by this, congratulated me on my efforts and sent me on my way. I felt very happy about the whole interaction. Maybe I made them pause for thought about their own relationship with drink? Unlikely . . . when we got to Seville one threw up on the platform. Anyway, the important thing was that I had been my authentic self and they had respected me for it.

'Speaking your truth' overlaps with this. It just means telling people the way you feel about things, irrespective of whether they can relate, empathise or even understand. I spent years hiding the fact that I suffered from anxiety, occasional bouts of depression and 'generalised barmy thought condition'. Why? Because I was ashamed and I thought I had no right to feel the way I did. I was worried that people might think I was exaggerating my problems. That I was looking for attention. That I was weak and self-pitying. But, ultimately, I knew how I felt. I didn't feel the need to justify or rationalise it. I didn't need explanations or solutions. I just needed to say these things out loud and lift the weight of them from my shoulders.

So what if some people couldn't understand? So what if how I felt didn't seem to quite make sense? It was my truth and I fucking spoke it. And by doing so I started upon a road to a happier, more fulfilling, more open-hearted life.

There was a time when I bristled at the very phrase 'mental health'. It sounded overblown and pompous. Sure, we all have ups and downs. But, for fuck's sake, there's no point making a song and dance about it. My grandma used to tell me, 'Always get straight out of bed in the morning before your mind gets to thinking. No good ever came from that.' But this was a woman who had lived through the Blitz and lost her husband to cancer when he was only in his fifties. Her oldest daughter (my auntie Celia) died of a heart attack in her forties. Grandma had resolved to suppress all the pain of these experiences in order to get through the rest of her life and I don't blame her. Her generation were specifically advised to leave their trauma unmentioned after the war. Back then, it was assumed that you could just forget bad things eventually if you ignored them long enough.

But my own experiences of depression, anxiety and addiction changed my perspective. By the age of forty I decided that trying to suppress or escape from my feelings wasn't ever going to work. I started the hard work of confronting and processing them. It was the right decision and has changed my life for the better.

Every day is a good day to remember that all of us have mental health and, just like physical health, it can fluctuate from time to time. Everyone lives with anxiety to one degree or another. Life is fast, intense and full of relentless assaults on our senses. Worry, fear and insecurity are everywhere, stoked by social media and twenty-four-hour news. Plus, the world economy has been in the shitter for over a decade. No wonder we're all shitting ourselves half the time.

Unlike most physical ailments, bad mental health is often invisible and usually difficult to explain. You can just wake up feeling shit sometimes and, occasionally, that feeling can hang around for a while and make life pretty tough. As someone who has enjoyed a generally happy life punctuated by the odd prolonged episode of being suffocatingly miserable, I know how tough it is to suffer in silence.

The first couple of times I experienced depressive episodes I kept my mouth shut about it because I was ashamed and scared. Ashamed because I thought I had no good justification for feeling the way I felt. And scared of how people would react if I owned up. I thought they would say I was weak or mental or whiny or entitled. I thought I was all of those things.

We're going back more than ten years here, when attitudes were different. This widespread chat about mental health just wasn't a thing yet. I assumed that I was the only thirty-something bloke in the world who was waking up terrified and full of self-hate every day. I didn't realise that struggling with poor mental health was as common as catching a cold in winter. And that just like catching a cold, you didn't need a justification for it. Sometimes it just happens. When it does, you need to recognise it and take care of yourself.

This is why I write and talk about this subject nowadays. I'm no expert on mental health, that's for sure. First and foremost, this is a selfish exercise: getting stuff off my chest makes me feel better. It's like a release valve on a pressure cooker. I like to normalise talking about the ups and downs of my mental health. Talking and writing about it helps me do that. The more I do it, the more casual it becomes, the less scary it is.

That's just what works for me. Not everyone is as comfortable with blurting out every detail of their inner lives. I don't blame them either and I'm not saying it is necessary for you to produce confessionals as publicly (and relentlessly) as I do. But even if it's just in conversation with people you trust, I think everyone should make themselves more comfortable with talking out loud about the way they feel. You don't have to make a massive deal out of it. Just be honest about the way you feel. Chuck it into conversation in a casual way. Normalise anxiety. It's just part of being human, after all.

Sharing with others helps you feel less alone (and a lot less weird) than you thought you were. People are kinder than you think when you show a bit of vulnerability. Sometimes, just having them quietly listen and understand can work wonders for your mood. And sometimes they can help you break your worries down, making them seem less overwhelming. They might even help you make a plan on how to make things better (even if that plan is simply to step back, take a breath and do nothing).

But perhaps the best reason for being a little bit more open about yourself is that it shows others that you might be up for them sharing back. By chucking the odd remark about your own struggles into conversation (something as small as 'I had a shit night's sleep, up all night worrying about everything and nothing again') you advertise yourself as an ally to others. They might pick up on something you said and realise you are someone they can open up to.

Sometimes people open up to me. I'm gutted for mates when they tell me they're going through a bad phase. But I am also touched that they feel they can talk to me about it.

It goes round and round in what marketing wankers call 'a virtuous circle'. I am forever grateful to the people who first understood me when I finally confessed to my own mental health struggles. And I try to show people around me that I am there if they ever need me. I'm no expert and I can't fix their problems. But I can at least listen, understand and tell them that things will definitely get better. They really will.

We're all in this together, gang.

Chapter 5

Stop Shitting Yourself
About Being Perfect

'High performance' is a term that used to be applied to cars but, nowadays, it is increasingly applied to human men.

There are a legion of hugely popular podcasts and social media accounts devoted to this cult of workaholism. They feature men who celebrate hyper-busyness and boast about their inability to ever relax. The word 'performance' is used in a very broad sense: almost every last aspect of existence is rendered a performance by these people. From getting up in the morning to breathing, thinking, eating, exercising, working and sleeping: our lives are carved up into a million and one micro-performances, each of which can be modified and fine-tuned to optimise outcomes. It is exhausting and probably doesn't do too much for the mental health of its acolytes.

If every second of your life is part of a continuous process of modification and improvement, there is little space left for rest, reflection, joy or leisure. It's all go, go, go in the world of high performance. It's as if the high-performing gang are preparing for the aftermath of an apocalypse in which we will all be required to practise elaborate survival techniques to survive. While the rest of us have just been spending our time eating crisps, stroking the cat, enjoying a movie and laughing at the beautiful absurdity of life, the high performers have been training themselves to problem-solve with razor-sharp mental precision, withstand immersion in sub-zero waters and reply to all of their emails before 5 a.m. These are the skills that will ensure that they are the ones whose optimised DNA serves as a launchpad for a new, improved human race while the rest of us lazy schlubs just die out. It sounds extreme but I truly believe that, if you really buy into all this high-performance stuff and follow it to its natural conclusion, it's all about cheating death, hacking evolution and crushing the weak as you do so.

There is a tedious self-importance to the advocates of high performance: an uptight seriousness that lacks charm and imagination, an obsession with dreary notions like 'consistency' and 'process' that represent the antithesis of almost everything that ever generates anything fun, interesting or artistic. More pertinently, I've seen many of its advocates go fucking mental. I should know because I have flirted with it myself.

At the start of 2016 I was newly sober and I decided I wanted to lose two stone and pay off all my debts by June. Relatively quickly, I was burning calories and making money like a lunatic and, by April, I had achieved both my goals way ahead of schedule. Was I happy? Well, yes, I'm afraid to tell you that I was. At least briefly. I was sober, slim and minted. I'm not going to tell you that those things don't feel great, especially when you first experience them.

I can tell you how I made it all happen so quickly. But, more importantly, I can explain why I came to regret everything about those mental few months.

The previous few years of my life had seen me give up exercise and financial prudence in favour of daytime drinking and cocaine use. As a result, I was fat and skint. But sobriety had provided me with a surfeit of energy that, back then, I didn't quite know how to channel. I put it all into becoming an extreme high performer (also known as a self-absorbed prick).

Having recently watched *Limitless* with Bradley Cooper (a film about a slob who takes a magic pill that turns him into an uber-productive superman) I envisaged a New Sam, who could achieve any goal he set himself, no matter how extreme or outlandish.

I started getting up at 5 a.m. to run by the river or train at the gym. I bought a NutriBullet and took to making myself putrid green juices for breakfast. I started hosting a daily radio show while simultaneously running my own production company. Yes, I was smashing my goals. But I was also insane. I was wild-eyed and jumpy. I was always amped up and, I think, pretty difficult to be around. I thought I was looking after myself because I looked healthier. But I had taken things to dangerous extremes and I was completely unable to relax. As a result, my moods fluctuated wildly; I lost my temper with people at work regularly in ways that surprised even me. I made rash decisions that weren't really aligned with my core values. Which is another way of saying that I acted like a bit of a wanker at times. I sacked people on a whim. I shouted when I didn't get things done the way I wanted. And when I was at home, I was always exhausted, grumpy and uncommunicative with my family. My wife had put up with the previous few years of inebriation. Now she must have felt like she was out of the frying pan and into the fire.

I had become enchanted by high-performance culture: the sort of psychopathic thinking that drives you to physical and mental extremes on the premise that any lesser goals represent failure. High-performance culture presupposes that it is impossible to be happy or comfortable with yourself unless you are constantly pursuing some objective form of excellence in everything you do.

I burned out completely when I tried to live that way. I alienated people who I loved and who loved me. I lost a few friendships. And, deep down, I wound up disliking myself. Not quite as much as I had disliked myself when I was drinking – but not far off. I had effectively replaced one set of manic addictions with another. The motivations were the same: I didn't feel as if I was enough. I needed outside validation. I wanted something to fill a void inside. But I was looking in the wrong places.

I didn't really want to be like Bradley Cooper's character in *Limitless*. He was, on reflection, a complete psychopath and a bit of a prick. Not much different from Patrick Bateman in *American Psycho*, or the wanker's wanker, Andrew Tate. They're all lunatics with probable daddy issues who want to prove to everyone, especially themselves, that they are better than everyone else.

I'm not trying to go all hippy on you here. I'm just saying that when we work together, accept each other's flaws, live with our own imperfections and try to empathise with others, we deliver great things. When we are locked in a constant state of competitiveness with ourselves and others, we generate a lot of anger and toxicity.

The Beatles were not big into high-performance culture when they made *Sgt. Pepper*. Picasso was not up at 5 a.m. on the green juice during his rose period. Aneurin Bevan was not skipping lunch or keeping an ambition journal when he founded the NHS. Beautiful things happen often when people are just at ease with themselves. Being comfortable in your own skin is what matters. I was never comfortable in my own skin when I was drinking or when I was in high-performance mode. It was only when I stepped back from all of that, reflected carefully on who I really wanted to be, what my values were and where all my low self-esteem was rooted, that I became a more balanced, happier person.

Now I exercise, I work, I earn and I play. But I am measured in everything I do. Crucially, I am not doing any of that stuff to create a false impression of success to myself or others. I do it to allow myself to focus on the things that I really love: spending time with my family, being creative, having fun and relaxing in my own small (often peculiar) ways.

I'm inclined to think that anyone who is immersing themselves in a life of constant distraction, whether that be drugs, drink, exercise, business or fucking crypto-trading, is not entirely comfortable in their own skin. Men are competitive by nature and often seem unable to assess their own value unless it is in comparison to their peers. It's a shame because that sort of individualistic, sharp-elbowed one-upmanship is pretty toxic. This thinking is a form of social Darwinism. It's inherently individualistic and ultimately opposed to the sort of connectedness, love and understanding that brings about most of the human race's best achievements.

Rather than teach high performance in schools, we should maybe be teaching balance: the art of calibrating life, work, play, rest, study and whatever else floats your boat, in such a way that you might be able to one day attain contentment. This is an ongoing challenge that all of us – high performers, low performers and all of us wishy-washy bastards in the middle – are engaged in every day. I am not there yet, but at least I know I am heading in the right direction, now I've quit all the green juice and 5 a.m. starts.

I saw an ad at a bus stop for a drink called Rockstar Energy. The slogan was 'Fuel the Do-It-All You'. It was plastered on the side of the shelter where my daughter waits for her bus to school. Presumably she is the target audience. Kids her age guzzle these drinks because they're told it will help them drag themselves in and out of school, get their studying done and still have the get-up-and-go to have fun with their mates. It's like their minds are being softened up to the cult of productivity before they even reach adulthood. Young people are told that they must study hard, play an instrument, get some work experience, help the elderly, participate in various sports clubs and learn to code before they've even tried their first fag.

What a load of horseshit. I don't make my kids do anything beyond going to school, doing their homework and reading the odd book once in a while. That's enough. Why would I want to exhaust the poor bastards any further? There is a mental health epidemic among young people in this country. I am not surprised: they are under obscene amounts of pressure to live out a demented, Thatcherite fantasy of what childhood should be. I reckon childhood should be balanced carefully between learning and lazing about.

They teach you important stuff at school, sure. But, when I was a kid, I'm convinced I learned an equal amount while lazing about, listening to records, reading comics and just thinking things through. Adolescence is a unique little window in life where your brain is ready to tackle some of life's bigger questions unencumbered by the dreary expectations of adulthood.

You can spend your time absorbing movies, music and books or just sitting about in your bedroom staring at the ceiling. You can hang about with your mates talking shit and doing absolutely nothing of consequence. It helps you to form your personality and develop a worldview. It nurtures the imagination. Plus, it's fun. You don't have to make decisions or shape responses based on scary practical matters like money or careers. You can just see where the wind takes you. The opportunity to do that stuff is brief, so it's worth making the most of. Fuck your Duke of Edinburgh and your viola lessons. Go up the park and dick around with your mates for a few hours or stay at home and watch reruns of the American *The Office*. It's good for the soul.

Productivity is an addiction like any other. We all get a nice little buzz from completing a task or reaching some benchmark of personal development. Nothing wrong with that. Unless you start to rely on those little buzzes as your only reliable source of comfort in an otherwise anxious existence. Before you know it, you are hooked on non-stop progress, achievement and growth. You need to be busy all the time. As you continually chase that buzz, you can become increasingly resistant to its impact. And so you require greater achievements, bigger successes, a more relentless schedule in order to maintain the same basic level of contentment.

There is very little difference between this and an addiction to booze, coke or meth. True, being busy might make you richer, fitter or smarter (although there's no guarantee – history is littered with as many lazy success stories as it is overactive losers). And you might argue that drugs and booze do the opposite: they make you poor, desperate and unhealthy. But even that's not strictly true. Cocaine can make you more productive in fleeting bursts. Alcohol, taken in the right amounts, can give you the sense of relaxed confidence that might well assist your endeavours socially, professionally and romantically. But they are short-term fixes for your state of inner discontent. The more you rely on them, the less you can cope with life naturally, without those stabiliser wheels.

Productivity addiction is just the same. If you can't learn to sit in a room content to be alive, enjoying your own company, coping peacefully with the ups and downs of your own thought patterns, then life is always going to be a frantic struggle. You're always going to be seeking a distraction. Can you stay busy and productive for ever and ever? Probably not. But you could certainly die trying.

Sometimes I feel as if my goal is to ascend to a distilled form of perfect laziness. I think that I will only be truly content when I have learned to do fuck-all for days on end without any sense of guilt, shame or worry. I am nowhere near that state yet. But at least I have ditched the strange, vaguely fascistic urge to be regarded as a constantly busy, do-it-all cyber-human.

This is what awful marketing people want us to dream of. They want us to buy their energy drinks and pursue the fool's gold of perma-activity. If we just learn to do fuck-all, then they would be screwed. We can't let stupid marketing people shape our dreams. We are all better than that. I mean, what possessed them to call their drink Rockstar Energy anyway? Rock stars are notoriously lazy. David Bowie and Prince didn't learn their trade by subscribing to online productivity courses. If Jimi Hendrix were still around today, it's doubtful he would be drinking energy pop, competing in triathlons or applying to be on *The Apprentice*. Rock stars learn how to be rock stars by staying out late at the disco then waking up at lunchtime the next day and spending the afternoon thinking idly about space or sex or God or nice clothes.

The spring I turned forty-seven I remember finishing my book, painting the bathroom and running 100 km in thirty days for charity. It felt great. But I couldn't sustain that level of achievement. Nor did I want to try. It would have been bad for me mentally, physically and emotionally. I thought about following it all up by having a personal 'Slob June'. Sit around in my pants all day, eating crisps, playing *FIFA* – that sort of vibe. But after a day or two of that, I'll admit, I started to feel a bit anxious and miserable.

Like everyone else, I have spent my whole life being indoctrinated into the cult of productivity. It's natural that I should feel weird when I try to take a break.

Someone once gave me a great bit of advice on how to seek balance: each day, try to do one thing that's productive and one thing that's relaxing. They can be small things. The key is to set the bar pretty low. If you start each day with a lengthy to-do list and don't complete it, you will probably feel crap about yourself. But if your list only has two things on it (and one of those things is a bit indulgent) then you've got a great chance of succeeding.

Mix it up. Maybe send an important work email in the morning then grab a twenty-minute nap in the afternoon. Or have a run, then read a book. Do the laundry then smoke a fag. Whatever works for you. It all comes down to personal circumstances and taste. The point is, try not to get too wrapped up in being busy all the time.

Peace is all I ever craved. But for many years I lived in a world where peace was impossible to find: society seemed to bombard me with goals to chase, ambitions to set, aspirations to fulfil. Career, money, love, family, home, health . . . every aspect of life was contaminated by a competitive culture that made things that should have been enjoyable feel like a brutal gladiatorial contest. Feelings of failure haunted me. Drink and drugs provided an apparently simple escape from those feelings.

I eventually managed to step out of all that and get some sensible perspective on life. But the ugly world of hyper-intense ambition still exists – and seems to be getting worse. The podcast charts are increasingly dominated by batshit shows presented by dead-eyed narcissists preaching hyper ambition.

This sort of thinking is rooted in a fundamentally right-wing worldview: the idea that everyone can succeed if they are just willing to work hard enough. It ignores all context: the myriad socio-economic, racial and other cultural obstacles to success. More dangerously, it works on an assumption that we all share one objective aim in life which is to be the absolute best at everything we do. This is the warped thinking of uptight psychopaths and not of happy, content, relaxed people. Most people want to learn to be comfortable with whatever life throws at them.

For fuck's sake, slow down. This sort of culture is dangerous. It sends its advocates barmy and it amplifies a message to young people that they are never enough. They have to strive, compete and graft incessantly to prove they are of value. It's all a bit Nietzschean, isn't it? I call it 'cocaine thinking': a state of mind that means you are constantly hyped up, never quite satisfied with anything and always fretting about where the next little hit is going to come from.

Ridding myself of that mindset was one of the most difficult but positive things I ever did. It takes a lot of hard work to realise just how stupid hard work really is.

We live in a world where Andrew Tate is wildly popular, particularly among young men. He is, of course, the symptom and not the cause of this lonely and pitiful brand of modern masculinity. It is a culture inhabited by young men who unironically talk and think like eighties action heroes: preoccupied with being dominant, powerful, perfectionists. They want to be seen as the best at everything they do: physically strong, mentally sharp, philosophically bold. Most of all, they want to be taken seriously. And that is the biggest shame of all.

At least when I was a young dickhead I knew I was a young dickhead. Like most lads of my generation, we were inspired just to have a laugh. We were inspired by happy-go-lucky types like footballing maverick Paul Gascoigne and snooker bad-boy Jimmy White, who seemed to have a healthy grasp on the fact that life was absurd and none of us have much control over its outcomes, so we all might as well have a laugh along the way. Which wasn't the best ideology to live by (Gazza was a drunk with a record of domestic abuse and Jimmy once admitted to getting so drunk that he stole the corpse of his brother from the undertakers and took it to the pub with him the night before the funeral) but I feel as if it was slightly sunnier than what Tate has to offer. It was certainly less bitter, angry and aggressive.

This attitude to life was also more human: by having a sense of our own irrelevance – a healthy notion of how fleeting and pointless life is – we were able to enjoy the moment. A really good foundation for all of this is to avoid seeing other men as your competitors and women as being an alien species. Accepting that we are all humans – and that the history of our civilisation shows that humans always seem to triumph when we establish connection and understanding – is a good starting point both for your own mental health and the future of our species. Just a thought – might be bollocks.

But the Tate outlook is about all those things: it is a warped interpretation of Darwinism, in which the strongest survive and all of us are in constant conflict. Not only is this scientifically inaccurate (evolutionary winners are the ones who learn to work together, not against each other) it is so unforgivably dull and joyless. Think about the best times you had at school: I bet you were laughing with your mates. You could sit through a hundred hours of Andrew Tate and his followers on TikTok or YouTube and not see any of them laugh once.

It's such a shame that the world has become so serious. You know who I blame? People. Before the internet, we weren't all exposed to the billions of other humans all over the world with their strange ideas, irritating habits or horrible opinions. Now, we are force-fed that stuff every day. No wonder young people are so angry and frustrated and confused. They are exposed constantly to a tsunami of human failure. It must make a lot of them feel angry and scared. The likes of Andrew Tate deliver a simplistic and palatable strategy for navigating their way through the shit. He's a plain old grifter and young male dickheads are his low-hanging fruit.

If we really want our kids to stop being groomed by online wankers, we just need to teach them to start laughing at things – starting with themselves.

When I was a kid I liked Madness frontman Suggs, *Grange Hill*'s top boy, Tucker Jenkins, and West Ham strikers Tony Cottee and Frank McAvennie. They were all young, successful, talented and free-thinking. As a teenager I liked Shaun Ryder from the Happy Mondays, Chuck D from Public Enemy, Prince, Eddie Murphy and Vic and Bob. I felt like there was a mild cockiness to them, like urchins made good by virtue of their flair and swagger. That was the sort of thing that appealed to me then and it still does now. These were positive role models: talented, fearless, authentic and cheeky. A great bunch of lads.

You need great men to look up to while you're building a personality for yourself. You spot things you like about blokes you admire and try to piece them all together, mix them up with your own experiences and mould it all into an identity of your own. During this process, you have to be careful not to look up to wankers. These days, that's more difficult than ever because – in the public eye at least – the wanker-to-good-bloke ratio seems to have fallen badly out of sync.

These thoughts might just be the embarrassing sputterings of a middle-aged bastard, of course, but I do worry that there are more wankers like Tate presenting themselves as role models these days. While Tate grew up working class, the aspirations he sells are elitist and superficial. There seems to be no celebration of fundamental human qualities or universal sources of contentment. His design for life is all about the acquisition of expensive supercars.

I've got teacher mates who say that Andrew Tate is a serious problem for them. The lads they teach genuinely love him, despite his toxic idiocy and despicable antics. They think he's great because he drives a Bugatti. My mate told his pupils that Tate was an arsehole and they replied, 'But sir, we've seen the old banger you drive to work in. Why would we believe your word over his?'

That's the problem. Late-stage capitalism, an elitist society, a homogenised culture and rampant consumerism have created a generation who are impressed by little more than displays of vast wealth and a boneheaded 'fuck you' attitude.

In 2023, Elon Musk and Mark Zuckerberg made an abortive attempt to fight each other in a cage in Las Vegas to settle their business disputes. It's the sort of thing *The Simpsons* would have made a joke about thirty years ago but it was actually happening: two billionaires who made money so quickly and easily that they never really needed to emotionally mature, fighting each other because they are permanently frozen in a state of adolescence.

I think I've raised my son well enough to understand that Tate is a wanker and the likes of Musk and Zuckerberg are, at best, dickheads. But even if he knows what men not to like, he still needs other men who he can actively look up to.

He did have Declan Rice, who was brilliant, funny and kind, and, crucially, played for West Ham. But then he signed for Arsenal and the one decent role model my son had is tainted for ever.

What young lads need is role models who can be brave, cool, funny, tough and all the other things our basest instincts aspire to be while also managing to be sensitive, kind, respectful and intelligent.

What they need is more Tucker Jenkins and less Andrew Tate.

David Goggins is a former member of the elite US military force the Navy SEALs, a motivational speaker and very much part of the high-performance brand of new masculinity. With his military background, his shtick is catnip to millions of blokes around the world who draw comparisons between warfare and their own relatively humdrum lives. And life can sometimes feel a bit boring. Sometimes it seems too easy. Rather than feel grateful for the safety and comfort of their lives, some men feel guilt and frustration. They buy into the idea that men are 'built' for more adventurous and dangerous endeavours like hunting, gathering, fighting and conquering. They don't appreciate that humankind's triumph is to find ways of evolving away from all that stuff.

Hunting, gathering, fighting and conquering sounds like a pain in the arse to me. I know sitting at a desk writing emails for a living can be dull, but it's surely better than having to go out in the cold to spend days stalking, capturing, killing then cooking a deer. The whole idea of man being genetically programmed to live the hunter-gatherer lifestyle is utterly spurious. It's the daft imaginings of men working overtime to romanticise their own existences. Yes, men once lived in caves and had to hunt for food. But that was a long time ago and, let's be honest, our ancestors were as thick as pigshit. We've moved on since then and have the know-how to live more civilised and convenient lives. Don't feel bad or embarrassed about it. Feel grateful that you're alive in the twenty-first century, with all its infrastructure, innovative farming techniques and domestic central heating. Get over this obsession with your cavemen ancestors. They were probably fucking boring to talk to anyway.

I sat next to a bloke at a wedding once who kept loudly boasting about the wilderness axe-craft course he had just completed. A weekend of fucking about with axes in the woods, carving bits of wood, making fires, chopping up small animals and so on. Absolutely disgusting if you ask me. He sensed I was unimpressed by his display of juvenile machismo, and so he challenged me: 'What would *you* do if you had to survive in the middle of nowhere with nothing but an axe? You'd be fucked.'

I had to admit, he was right. I absolutely would be fucked. There are millions of other far-fetched scenarios he could have quizzed me about in which I would have been fucked too: stuck up a mountain with an egg whisk; stranded on Mars with nothing but a banjo. I'll be the first to admit that I am wholly unprepared for these sorts of situations. To be honest, I'd struggle to put up a two-man tent at a music festival. But I figure the chances of any of these things ever happening to me are so remote (even camping at a festival is something I feel I am very unlikely to ever do again) that it's not really worth me taking the time and energy to prepare for them. I'm much better off doing stuff that helps me in real life, like learning to cook using the array of utensils in my kitchen or submitting my tax returns in a timely manner. Fantasies about post-apocalyptic survival used to be the stuff of children's adventure comics but, these days, are the basis of popular podcasts and books created by serious academics and scientists and devoured by grown men. It's all a bit fucking weird. I wish men were able to feel happy with the actuality of their lives and didn't have to seek meaning in ludicrous daydreams about their supposed warrior instincts.

All of that said, Goggins has a trademark motivational concept that I think is really brilliant. He calls it 'The Cookie Jar'. In his mind, there is a jar in which he keeps all the successes and failures he has ever experienced. When times get tough and he starts to feel shit about himself, he reaches into this jar and pulls out an example of something he has overcome in the past. Maybe it was a break-up, a financial blow or career setback. Sometimes, he says, it's something broader, such as the racial abuse he has received throughout his life.

Whatever it is, it serves as a powerful reminder that he has overcome shit in the past, so he will do so again. And each time he does it, he will become stronger.

As Goggins puts it: 'Remind yourself of how badass you are in times of need.'

I was introduced to this thought by my personal trainer, Jordan. He applies it to physical fitness: the idea that when you're struggling to run that extra mile or lift that extra kilo, you can reach into the cookie jar to remind yourself that you have done it before. You tell your body that there is nothing to be afraid of and that you know you are capable. It can apply to any sort of challenge.

In recent years, as I have tried to come to terms with a new way of living, I have faced my share of challenges. An economic crisis triggered by the incompetent and mercifully short-term prime minister, Liz Truss, sent my mortgage repayments spiralling almost beyond the point of affordability. I had to contemplate the prospect of losing my home while also going through the process of shutting down a business, managing to keep up with my day-to-day work to make ends meet and just the general obligations of being a husband and father. None of it was uniquely challenging: these are the occasional struggles of the privileged, middle-class, developed countries. But still, it sucked. There were times when it all felt overwhelming. In the past, that sort of overwhelm might have driven me to the comforting oblivion of drink and drugs. But these days I have two safety nets that stop me from burning out and doing something stupid.

Firstly, I recognise the stress and exhaustion I am feeling and acknowledge the need to take some time out to rest. In the past, I would have just kept ploughing on to the point of collapse.

Second, I have my cookie jar. When I felt that the financial worries or business challengers were going to drag me under, I recalled the tougher times I had navigated my way through in the past. I'd faced worse. I'd got through worse. I was equipped to do it all again. Things are a lot easier when you believe in yourself. We all have our own jars. The fact that we are all here today means that we've managed to face down all the crap life has thrown at us so far and lived to tell the tale. It's all there in the cookie jar. Or, as we Brits prefer to call it, the biscuit tin.

Next time you're having a shitty day, have a dip inside yours.

Chapter 6

Stop Shitting Yourself About Work

Between the ages of four and fourteen I shared a bedroom with my brother Cas, who is seven years older than me.

There was an informal border down the middle of the room. On my side, there were torn-out pictures from *Shoot* magazine stuck to the wall, jumbled toys spilling from shelves and West Ham ephemera draped everywhere (he was a QPR fan but just had to put up with it). His side was completely bare, like the rarely used pied-à-terre of a travelling salesman. He had nothing on the walls and, seemingly, no personal possessions beyond a few items of clothing he would keep crumpled on the floor.

I thought he was a bit of a bully because, sometimes, he would lock me in the airing cupboard. But who could blame him? He was trying to blossom into a fully functioning adult while encumbered by a snot-nosed pipsqueak who was always playing with *Star Wars* figures on the carpet. Whenever Cas was diligently working his way towards third base with his latest squeeze, I would charge into the room clutching my plastic Millennium Falcon and making 'beow-beow' laser noises. On reflection, I would probably have locked me in the airing cupboard too.

Yes, we fought and argued. But he was my big brother and, while I'd never tell him to his face (not then, not now, not ever) I thought he was amazing. A charismatic hedonist who always had loads of girlfriends and rarely bothered going to school – what wasn't there to admire? To me, he was like Robin Hood.

Cas always had a job on the go: first a milk round, then selling hot dogs at QPR home games, then working as an usher at Hammersmith Odeon where he got paid to watch a different band play every night. He left school at sixteen but by the time he was seventeen he already had a glamorous job making adverts at a place in the West End. He never seemed to stop grafting. At least that's the way I saw it. I got the impression that if I wanted to live life by my own rules – like he did – I would have to learn to hustle and put a proper shift in.

I'm worried that my own kids don't have the same sort of role model in their lives. I mean, I do work pretty hard, I suppose, but it's just not very visible. I write and I broadcast. The problem is you can do all that from home these days. As far as my kids can see, I just sit about the house all day playing on my laptop. And yet, somehow, there is a roof over their head and food on the table. Plus, they each have their own bedroom.

I don't want them to fetishise the idea of hard work. Graft can only get you so far – my brother and I have both had our share of luck along the way. Some people work their balls off their whole life, but the odds remain stubbornly stacked against them. In the final analysis, work sucks, rest is awesome and capitalism is a rigged game. All I want to teach my kids is what Cas taught me: that you can do it on your own terms and have a laugh along the way.

I'll be the first to accept that my smooth, soft, beautiful hands have barely done a day's manual or 'proper' work in their life. But I don't make any apologies for that either. It was perhaps a couple of hours into my first shift as a milkboy, aged nine, when I decided that physical graft was not for me. And so I set about working out how to do something for a living that I actually enjoyed. The thing I always enjoyed most was mucking about. And I am proud to have identified various ways of monetising it over the past few decades. So what? It would have been easier for me to have found a boring job. I didn't want that. I liked coming up with ideas. I liked writing. I was good at talking. I enjoyed making people laugh. I decided that I would try to get paid for doing stuff like that. The trick was to come up with ideas so strong that people would pay to engage with them (if you have paid to read this book, then thanks for the money and the validation. If you borrowed it from a mate or nicked it from a shop, then I suppose I am still somewhat grateful). I feel lucky, yes. But just because I don't have calluses all over my hands doesn't mean I haven't worked hard along the way.

I received my first ever creative commission when I was eleven years old. I was keen on drawing cartoons at the time. I copied characters out of the *Beano, Roy of the Rovers* and Marvel comics, trying to perfect a bunch of different styles. I had dreams of becoming a professional illustrator when I grew up. My brother Dom had a girlfriend who worked as a care assistant in a home for kids with disabilities. She said she'd pay me twenty quid to make some flashcards featuring famous Disney characters such as Mickey, Donald, Goofy and all the rest. It was for some sort of educational game.

I was excited about the prospect of getting paid to draw. But I kept putting it off and putting it off until the deadline day arrived and she was on her way round to collect the finished work. In a panic, I grabbed some pieces of typing paper and a ballpoint pen and attempted to draw Mickey Mouse from memory. It was shit. Tried Donald and it was even worse. I decided my only option was to trace the images but the only Disney pictures I had were on some old novelty pants. So there I was, twenty minutes before the client showed up, sat at the kitchen table, trying to trace pictures of Mickey Mouse off a pair of pants onto a piece of A4 typing paper. What a shambles.

When my brother's girlfriend arrived, I handed her the work shamefully but still had the balls to ask if I'd get paid. At this point Dom intervened with a long, humiliating lecture about my slipshod attitude. I'd had weeks to get this sorted, he pointed out. I should have sourced some images of the characters, practised sketching them and then got hold of some proper materials with which to make the cards. I had been lazy, disorganised and shit. He insisted that his girlfriend didn't give me a penny. He was absolutely right. His lecture was so powerful and accurate that it has lived with me ever since.

While my mates were topping up their pocket money by delivering newspapers in the cold and dark, I had been given the chance to earn some dough out of doing something fun that I would have otherwise done for free. And I had wasted the opportunity. I had fucked it up. I was a worthless piece of entitled shit. Dom didn't actually say those last bits. I added them in myself and still do so to this day, whenever I feel as if I have failed to produce something to the standard I deem acceptable.

The shitshow of my first ever commission still haunts me. Dom has probably forgotten about it by now. I'm sure his ex-girlfriend has too (yes, they split up a few months later and I have always wondered if my professional incompetence might have played some part in that).

Beating yourself up over a lack of productivity is common to us all. I think my brother taught me some important lessons back then that have served me well over the years. But I also think I have dwelled on them too much at times. Professionalism is important, I guess. But the need to be constantly producing, delivering, improving and perfecting is dangerous and addictive. It's one thing resolving to do the work you've promised to do on time and to a decent standard. It's another thing to start hating yourself every afternoon when you realise that only four items on your overly ambitious thirty-item to-do list have been crossed off.

Life just can't be about constant progress. We are, all of us, participants in a constantly oscillating game of one step forwards, two steps back. Consistency is an overvalued concept. It means doing things the same way every day in the hope that we will slowly achieve improved results. Which sounds fucking boring, doesn't it?

Life goes up, life goes down. Sometimes you win, sometimes you don't. Some days, you might wake up full of beans, go for a run, smash out a load of work, hit all your deadlines and be home in time to knock up a delicious meal for your family. Other days you just feel inexplicably nauseous and knackered, get fuck all done, order the kids pizza for tea and fall asleep in front of *Question Time* consumed by a sense of self hatred.

A lot of men have become enchanted with applying the stratagems and protocols of elite athletes to their everyday lives. But not all of us are elite athletes. Most of us are just dreary corporate slaves. We are not all built with the same inclinations as those exceptional sportsmen who are able to achieve constant improvement every single day of their lives. They are referred to as 'elite' for a reason. It is not healthy for average folk to apply the same standard to themselves. You will be left with a constant sense of failure. You don't have to end every day by checking off everything on your to do list. You don't even need a fucking to-do list.

You don't need to be in a state of perpetual progress to be happy. Sometimes you can be perfectly content just sitting still, doing nothing and letting the bullshit of your mind swirl around a bit. Feel sad, learn to live with it, understand it will pass and tomorrow might be more fun.

Life is not a race; it's much more nuanced than that. And more enjoyable too. Races are a pain in the arse.

When I was eighteen, I was a passionate Labour Party member and managed to get some unpaid work experience at the House of Commons, running errands for the MP for Peckham, Harriet Harman. It was a real privilege to be exposed to that world at such a young age, one year before I went off to study politics at university. The older I get the more I realise how lucky I was. Labour was still in opposition back then and Harriet Harman was Shadow Chief Secretary to the Treasury. I learned a lot and she was a great boss.

But, to be honest, I was a bit of a sulky and unappreciative dickhead half the time. I was only paid my expenses and I actually resented having to go into the office every day when all of my unemployed mates were sitting around at home, playing video games and smoking weed. I just didn't like having to go into the same place at the same time every day. Mind you, Harriet did insist that I only ever worked a four-day week, telling me that I needed to 'spend my Fridays buying guitar strings, or whatever it is teenagers do these days'.

The office was on Millbank, the long road that runs alongside the Thames next to Parliament. We shared a department with Gordon Brown and Peter Mandelson. My fellow researchers included Ed Balls, Yvette Cooper and Ed Miliband, older and much more senior than me. Miliband was a good bloke who was dead clever but didn't mind talking to me about football when he realised that was the only thing I was capable of showing any enthusiasm for. He got to write speeches and draw up policy documents for Harriet. I made tea, did the photocopying and ferried documents between offices, skulking about Westminster with my Sony Sports Walkman plugged permanently into my ears.

One evening Harriet gave me a draft copy of a speech she was due to deliver at that week's Treasury Questions session in the Commons. She'd be up against her governmental rival, Michael Portillo. It was a big deal. I was to take the speech that night to one of her Parliamentary colleagues for his perusal and comments. Only I forgot to do so and went to an evening match at West Ham with the draft still in my rucksack. On the way to the game, I met up with my pals at our usual haunt, a pub called the Grave Maurice on the Whitechapel Road. A former HQ of the Krays, it was a rough-and-tumble sort of place, particularly on match days. A couple of pints into the pre-match refreshments,

I produced the speech from my bag and waved it about, trying to show my mates how important I was. Naturally, none of them gave a shit.

When we headed for the stadium, I absent-mindedly left the speech on a beer-sodden table. I only realised this twenty minutes later when I was about to enter Upton Park. I probably should have gone straight back to the pub to retrieve it. But I was lazy, stupid and drunk so I just called the Grave Maurice from a payphone, asked a barman to have a look around for the speech, which hadn't been destroyed or stolen.

But even after the match I didn't bother going back to the pub. I left it to the next day to collect the speech, which by then was rippled and brown from dried lager and fag ash. I binned it and told Harriet that I had simply forgotten to deliver it. She didn't have to know about its detour through the pubs of east London and had another copy of the speech which she used in the Commons that afternoon. I chose to believe the whole incident was chalked off as an 'all's well that ends well' sort of thing. But my casual approach to matters of political sensitivity was probably noted by the higher ups in the Labour party. Hey ho.

All I know is that Harriet became deputy prime minister and the researchers I used to count as drinking pals became government ministers, while I was editing a showbiz gossip magazine. It's funny how life turns out, but I suppose my slapdash attitude was never likely to propel me up the political ladder.

Mind you, it wasn't just politics that was the problem. In almost every job I've ever had, I've been reluctant to put the work ahead of my personal affairs. When I was young and working my way up, I hated the way that bosses told me what to do and where to be. I resented having to work more hours than I was being paid for, just to prove that I was 'hungry'. Then, when I became the boss, I hated the fact that I was expected to give up even more time and energy to work in return for the big salary and fancy title. Even when I had my own business, I didn't like the way that work occupied my mind at evenings and weekends, when I should have been focusing exclusively on fun stuff like family, friends and the *Police Academy* movies.

For many years, the way I coped with these occupational frustrations was to drink heavily. Guzzling booze to numb the pain of exhausting work patterns is no way to live.

Did my reluctance to follow rules and keep my head down make me unprofessional? No. Did it, in fact, make me more in touch with my natural human instincts? Possibly. Was leaving that speech in the boozer when I went to watch West Ham a sackable offence? Definitely.

Hard work can be a reward in itself. And even when it's not you just have to get on with it. But keeping half an eye on balance and reminding yourself and others around you that there is more to your life than graft is essential to staying sane.

My best ever boss was Phil Hilton, who gave me my break in journalism and used to tell me, 'I don't care when you get the work done or where you get it done. As long as you get it done on time and that it's good.'

Of course, I know that advice doesn't work in every job. I mean, you couldn't say that to a bus driver or a surgeon. But the principle of his words was important: they made me feel trusted, responsible and respected. They made me feel like a human being and an adult, which is the least any employee deserves.

Phil was the editor of *Men's Health* magazine, where I got my first job in journalism. This was 1997, when lads' mags still sold by the millions and the hedonistic culture they espoused prevailed among most young men. *Men's Health*, a British version of an equally successful US magazine, was a lone voice on the newsstand, encouraging men to drink in moderation, go to the gym regularly and be nice and sensitive towards the significant women (or men – there was a large gay readership) in their lives.

I loved working there. It hadn't been my first choice, of course. I knew nothing about exercise, moderation or sensitivity and would have been a lot more comfortable among the unreconstructed editorial teams at *Loaded* or *FHM*. But the only contact I had in the whole publishing business happened to be Phil, a mate of my brother's ex-girlfriend. He was kind enough to give me some advice on becoming a journalist and, eventually, gave me some work experience which later morphed into paid employment.

I learned a great deal about magazines from the smart, kind people who worked there. I started to learn a bit about healthy living too. I'd just spent three years as a layabout, drug-addled student who thought one game of five-a-side every month represented a more than adequate concession to personal fitness. Within a couple of months of writing articles about proper nutrition and abdominal crunch techniques, I was obsessed. I became really immersed in the importance of a low-fat diet (the big thing at the time) and exercising every day. I got really skinny and started to become a bit of a bore about it, to be honest. My girlfriend had to be very patient as I lectured her every night about the nutritional content of the pasta we had knocked up for dinner. I would waste whole lunch hours fretting over what you buy in the food section of Boots. I became that nutter you see earnestly examining the ingredients label on the side of a sandwich box.

Even though I was six-foot-two and only ten-and-a-half stone (which, looking back, sounds anything but healthy) I went to the gym every day and ran for ages on the treadmill to burn off what I had eaten. Writing this down now, I'm beginning to realise it all sounds a bit like I had some sort of disorder. Maybe I did. But, whatever, the main point is that I had fallen under the spell of a self-help organisation – which happened to be the magazine I was working for – and it had made my life complicated, stressful and tedious.

I should say that nobody on *Men's Health* meant for the advice on its pages to be anything other than sensible and handy. It was not an indoctrination scheme. There was no agenda other than to convey reasonable and well-researched advice in a fun and compelling way to people who were already interested in that sort of thing.

And yet I became spellbound by every word. I felt compelled to follow its teachings to the letter. The vibe of *Men's Health* was relaxed and benign, but I interpreted it as a militant call to arms. I was like one of those Christian fundamentalists in the Deep South who takes the easy-going vibes of the New Testament and turns it into a fire-and-brimstone attack on homosexuality and abortion rights.

Why did I allow myself to get so dangerously hypnotised by words that were never meant to cause anyone any harm? Maybe because I was young, impressionable and at a crossroads in my life. I felt anxious about the future and unsure of myself. Perhaps I was on the lookout for a set of rules to guide me: a roadmap for successful living that I could submit to. That sort of self-help guide can be so seductive when you're feeling vulnerable: it tells you that if you just trust the process you will succeed and find happiness. All you want is for the random factors to be removed from your life. A well-phrased guidebook can convince you that it's all so possible.

Men's Health is still going strong today and – in the current context of modern masculinity – seems more moderate than ever. But now, in the same space, we have a million influencers, lifestyle gurus and good old-fashioned grifters harnessing the might of social media to deliberately target the confused and vulnerable with advice and guidance that is ten times more manipulative and ten times less credible than the stuff we used to write. This is how we get a generation of young men hanging on the words of dreary, humourless men like the Canadian academic Jordan Peterson, with their charmless and angry brand of self-improvement advice.

I started to listen to the audiobook of *Atomic Habits* by James Clear a few months ago. I was running (slowly, crappily, pleasurably) by the river as I listened to his introduction, in which he explained, pretty compellingly, that every tiny decision we make from the moment we wake up in the morning has the capacity to change our life for the better. Every. Fucking. Decision.

The side of the bed you get out of. The speed with which you don your slippers. The route you take from the bedroom to the bathroom. The way you shake off your willy after finishing your morning piss. The technique with which you wash your hands. The brand of soap you use to wash them with. The size of towel you use to dry them off. Unless you choose not to dry them at all. Maybe there is a study showing 78 per cent of successful CEOs never dry their hands after washing because the dampness encourages them to type faster while replying to important business emails?

Once you start worrying about this shit, it's difficult to stop.

It might well be true that all decisions can be 'optimised' in order to improve 'performance'. But how can you possibly live your life in any sane, enjoyable or manageable way if you are subjecting every last micro-moment to this level of rumination?

The concept filled me with dread and made me think, If every single decision has the ability to make things better, it also has the ability to make things worse. In which case, I cannot afford to do anything, from take my first breath of the day to wipe the sleep from my eyes, without potentially setting off a chain of events that culminates in disaster. I choose the wrong motion with which to clean my teeth and suddenly – BANG – my kids are living in foster care and I'm in the Scrubs on a four stretch for public indecency. Fuck that. It doesn't bear thinking about.

This is all a bit rich coming from some bloke who is writing a book about mental health, granted. But, as I always try to emphasise, nothing I write here (or anywhere else) is supposed to be advice. Rather, it should be taken as the experiences and reflections of an average bloke who you may or may not be able to relate to. At the most, this is all supposed to let you know that you're not the only one dealing with life's bullshit. And that things can get better. After all, look at me: I eventually ended up leaving *Men's Health* and now I'm a full-time podcaster who just ate a fried-egg sandwich for his lunch. Truly, I am living the dream.

Just have a little faith in the future and in yourself. Don't examine the ingredients label on your supermarket sandwich. And don't fret too much about your morning routine. Know who you want to be; establish some broad values you believe in and try to stick to them; try not to be a cunt and don't sweat the small stuff. Sometimes, just try to switch off and use the force. Thinking too carefully about the potential outcomes of every decision you make is a recipe for acute anxiety disorder.

Most of all, try to steer clear of men on the internet dishing out advice. Including me.

In January 2003, non-league Farnborough Town played Arsenal, the Premier League champions, in the fourth round of the FA Cup at their tiny stadium in Hampshire. I was working as a Channel 5 news reporter for ITN at the time and had been dispatched to Farnborough the day before the game to do a story about it.

I had never intended to work as a bloke on the evening news, standing somewhere cold and rainy, talking bollocks into a handheld microphone. But that's what I had found myself doing in my mid-twenties. I'd first landed a job as host of my own weekly youth culture show but it had been cancelled after twelve months and I had to accept the channel's offer of work on the daily news bulletins. It felt a bit more grown-up than sitting in a studio interviewing pop stars in my jeans and trainers. Suddenly, I was wearing a suit and tie and working long shifts.

I'd get up in the morning and head into the studios on Gray's Inn Road, where I would scour the papers for stories to pitch in the morning meeting. If I was lucky, I'd get to nip round the corner to Westminster and interview a politician or cover a protest. If I was less lucky, I would have to jump in a van with a grumpy cameraman and dash off to somewhere in the provinces to cover something 'quirky' (like the bloke who was still driving around in a

Sinclair C5 twenty years after they'd been discontinued) or something plain boring (like the summer's day I was sent to Brighton to cover the fact that it was particularly hot. I had to put together two three-minute reports on that story, plus conduct a live, two-way conversation with the anchor, Kirsty Young, who was back in the studio. 'What's happening, Sam?' 'Well Kirsty, what can I say? It's boiling fucking hot . . .').

It was interesting work that got me out and about, paid OK and taught me how to put together compelling stories on the fly. Until I started in TV, I'd been working on monthly magazines, which allowed you to fuck about and get drunk for three-quarters of the month before squeezing all the work into the final week. The world of news reporting was rather more demanding.

I did well enough to earn a contract and the strange title 'Anti-War Correspondent' in the build-up to the invasion of Iraq in March 2003. It was my job to cover the huge protest campaign that erupted in the UK, with a neutral curiosity. I spent time on marches, interviewing activists and sometimes being shouted at by militant peaceniks who considered all journalists to be puppets of the military–industrial complex. I mostly had the utmost respect for the determined and passionate protesters I came across but I also had to tell a few hippies to fuck off along the way.

Anyway, back to Farnborough's Arsenal match. I inter-viewed some fans and employees of the club and knocked out the edit in the back of the camera van, then beamed it back to HQ via the massive satellite dish that sat on the vehicle's roof. These were wild times, before you could send that stuff around the world in seconds using Wi-Fi. By the time I got back to London, it was eight-ish. I was coming off the back of an eleven-day run of twelve-hour shifts. I was freelancing on the side too, writing about music for the *Guardian* and the *NME*. I interviewed everyone from Air and LCD Soundsystem to Girls Aloud and Kylie. It was fun, but it never stopped and I was exhausted without realising it. And whenever I wasn't working, I was drinking.

I was saying 'Yes' to anything and everything that came my way. I was doing it for three reasons: firstly, I was hyper-aware of how brilliant this sort of work was and how lucky I was to get the chance to do it. Who was I to turn anything down? Secondly, the money was decent. Not enough to make me rich but I was young, freelance and renting a slightly-too-expensive flat with my girlfriend, so I needed all the dough I could lay my hands on. Then, as now, I assumed that each bit of work I got offered would be my last; I was never confident enough to turn stuff down. Which brings me to my third reason: I did all this work because I couldn't countenance the idea of ever being exhausted. I thought I could do anything. I just thought it was normal to work ceaselessly without any concern for my own welfare. It's what everyone else seemed to do. My family and my friends and everyone else I could see around me: everyone just worked, worked, worked – only ever stopping to get pissed.

It was relentless: a completely insane regimen of graft that stretched the body and mind to breaking point. We all held ourselves together with alcohol and drugs to numb out the sense of dread, of being overwhelmed and of anxiety that hovered menacingly in the background. I am knackered just thinking about it.

When I got back from Farnborough I met my girlfriend at a mate's birthday party in a bar in west London. I had four or five bottles of lager then announced myself too tired to carry on and got a cab back home. Once there, I took two paracetamol, some antibiotics I'd been prescribed for the sore throat that had been haunting me for months and then I threw up in the sink. Next, I staggered into the bedroom, collapsed on the floor and had a violent epileptic seizure. As I came round, pissing all over my jimmy-jams, my girlfriend explained what had happened and suggested I go to bed, which I did. But five minutes later, I had a second fit, even more violent than the last. An ambulance was called; I had a third seizure on the way to hospital and then a fourth while lying on a gurney in A&E.

I stayed in that hozzy for the whole weekend, undergoing tests. I remember an elderly Indian man in the bed opposite telling me that I needed to slow down, sleep more and (and this is a verbatim quote because it has lived with me ever since) 'always carry a packet of Mini Cheddars around in your pocket' to stave off the jitters.

It was all excellent advice, of course. But I was twenty-six and wrote it off as the daft ramblings of a neurotic codger. Even when the doctor told me that the blood tests suggested I was suffering from exhaustion and needed to change my lifestyle, I nodded and feigned concern but secretly resolved there and then to ignore his advice. What a boring dickhead, I thought to myself. Doesn't he know that living like this is great fun?

I'm not sure, in retrospect, I was having much fun at all. I didn't have much of a plan for my career: I was just rolling with the punches, taking anything that came my way irrespective of whether it brought me any sense of fulfilment or satisfaction. I drank copious amounts of lager every night and the only food that passed my lips was takeaway or microwaved ready-meals. I played five-a-side football once a week and thought that was enough to keep me fit. I smoked weed to help me get to sleep; in those days, cocaine was still just an occasional weekend treat. I stumbled into bed every night in a state of complete inebriation before waking up a few hours later and starting the insane routine all over again. Like I say, none of this behaviour seemed abnormal at the time. Everyone I knew seemed to live this way. How are any of us still alive? Lucky, I guess.

As far as I am aware, there are fewer young people living the sort of draining, reckless and often unhappy lives that we lived back in the noughties. They seem to be more aware of what's good for them and stricter about setting boundaries to preserve their own mental and physical health. People moan about young people in the workplace being less willing to stretch themselves these days. But I think it's great. I don't want my kids to live their twenties the way I lived mine. There is a way of doing fun, interesting work of value without sacrificing your wellbeing. Sometimes you need to work hard to get where you're going. But the important thing is to understand the toll that hard work can take and add a bit of balance to your life. At the very least, when things are getting a bit intense at work, try eating properly and getting some decent kip. Going out on the piss all the time is not a sustainable means of unwinding. My generation was just hoodwinked by a conspiracy that told us overwork was the only way of fulfilling our dreams.

These days I focus on three things to make sure I stay well: sleep, strength and sobriety. All the science tells us that getting consistent, high-quality sleep is the secret to longevity, a sharp mind and healthy body. I prioritise good sleep over almost everything else. I get to bed at ten every night and, whenever possible, try to squeeze a cheeky kip into the middle of the day too. Basically, I fucking love sleep. It's my favourite hobby.

I lift weights to keep my body strong. Fitness experts reckon lifting weights is life's 'cheat code': it's not necessarily about looking jacked (I don't); it's about making your body more resilient. It's changed my life. I run – but for shorter distances and at a slower pace than I used to. I do so regularly, mostly for the sense of mental tranquillity it offers me.

As for sobriety: I couldn't do any of this other stuff if I was drinking. Alcohol fucks with your sleep quality, diminishes your physical strength and makes you too lazy to do the stuff that really makes you healthy and happy. I think booze and drugs deprive you of any peace, encourage shitty decisions and only cover up misery temporarily before bringing it back, even stronger, the next morning.

I'd have been well advised to adopt some of these habits in my twenties, but if someone had told me to focus on sleep, strength and sobriety back then I'd have pissed myself laughing. Instead, I just kept on pissing myself from epilepsy.

Life is brilliant. I'm happy to still be living it. And I always try to keep a packet of Mini Cheddars to hand.

I've been a self-employed gun-for-hire for the best part of my twenty-six-year career. I prefer the freedom and variety of being a freelancer. But it hasn't always been easy, especially in terms of my mental health. Working for yourself can be a minefield of insecurity, paranoia and loneliness. When I look back on my worst episodes of depression, anxiety and addiction, it's clear that work and money were often significant factors.

It took me more than twenty years to work out how to emotionally manage freelance life. As I edge towards fifty I think I've almost nailed it. It took me a long time but I think I worked out how to be creatively fulfilled, financially stable, relaxed, happy and not (very) insane.

In my opinion, success as a freelancer has nothing to do with process, daily routine, personal branding, refining your pitches or any of the other dreary bollocks you can read endless articles about on spurious career blogs. It's about perspective: working out exactly what you want out of your career and precisely how you want to balance it with the other parts of your life.

When I first went freelance in 2001, it wasn't out of choice. I'd taken a job at a start-up in the first digital bubble of the century. The company had gone bust after six months and I was left on my arse. But instead of thinking, *Oh fuck, I have had the desperate and precarious state of a freelancer imposed upon me,* I thought: *Great, now I can go freelance and live life on my own terms.* It was all about my mindset. You can see change as a bad thing or an opportunity.

Because I had fantasised about this life for the past five or six years, I had done some subconscious planning. I knew who I wanted to work for, I'd thought through how I might pursue the work and – perhaps most importantly of all – I had nurtured an identity in my imagination. I felt comfortable in my own mind that I could make a busy, diligent and dynamic freelancer.

It's not that I simply managed to 'manifest' a freelance career. With few contacts and not much time to make a success of it before the bailiffs knocked around, I hustled hard. I cold-called editors, pitched ideas non-stop and didn't read too much into it when I was ignored or knocked back. I didn't let little failures and false starts kill my ambition. I maintained my self-belief and knew that if I kept knocking on doors, people would eventually let me in.

All these years later I still have a similar approach to freelance work but I have tried to temper my tendency to work non-stop. Back then, I thought any time off represented a waste. Now, I realise how crucial down time really is.

When they first go freelance, lots of people get worried about the risk of falling to pieces, forgetting to shave and sitting in front of the telly all day eating cereal. They think that, without a corporate overlord cracking a whip, they will not be sufficiently incentivised to stay focused and professional. They are so scared that they self-impose ultra-strict regimens, with early morning starts at the desk/kitchen table, strictly assigned tea breaks and intimidating to-do lists.

Yes, it's quite good to impose a bit of discipline on yourself. But I always found that the prospect of not being able to pay my bills or feed myself was enough to stop me from sitting around in my dressing gown all day. I have never had any savings or parental safety nets. I realise now that the precarious nature of my existence was a real strength: it gave me focus and drive. It was what recovering alcoholics call 'the gift of desperation'. I had no option but to find paid work.

But I also understood that being self-employed was a privilege and that it was important to make the most of that. What was the point of being freelance if you were going to graft the same long hours as the worker bees and deny yourself the opportunities for leisure and relaxation it provides? I figured that I was saving an hour or two on daily commutes to dismal offices; I could afford to have leisurely breakfasts at a cafe, reading the paper, gathering my thoughts and generating ideas. That's the whole point of being freelance, especially in the creative industries. Freedom and down time are the catalysts for invention. Make use of them. No one ever came up with their best ideas sitting at a desk staring at a wall.

If you don't have a looming deadline or anything else that is an emergency, down tools and go to the cinema. Or read a book. Take a walk. Do all the stuff you dreamed of doing more of when you were a corporate slave. It's not lazy or negligent to do this. It counts as work. All the time you are living life in an enjoyable way you are enriching your mind and sparking your imagination.

You might think that empty time between deadlines is when you should be pitching and hustling: making contacts, firing off emails, nurturing your presence on social media.

But what you might not realise is that you are always hustling even when you're not. Everything you have done in your career is silently contributing to your next job, somewhere in the background. The work you've done, the people you've met, the jobs you've pitched for and just missed out on: it all counts. You exist in people's minds already. If your work has been good it will reward you at some point in the future.

I keep those points in my thoughts when I go for walks with the dog in the middle of the day, my phone switched off in my pocket. You don't always have to be 'on'. And in fact, being 'off' can serve you better. The best things tend to arrive when you are patient and a little ambivalent. Personally, my worst struggles have always been during periods when I was trying to force things. Pitching relentlessly, chasing answers, banging on doors: very often, when you get that frantic, you let your quality control slip. You say 'Yes' to any old shit just because you want to keep busy.

That said, I know it's hard to be measured when your back is to the wall. And you may well be reading this thinking, It's OK for you, you've been in the game for years and can afford to take it easy. First of all, I can't afford to do that. Yes, I have more experience and contacts than I had twenty years ago but I also have bigger bills to pay and more dependents to feed. Like I say, I have never saved a penny. I've no idea how people can afford to, to be honest. I've lived in London my whole life, where money is just absorbed the moment it lands in your account.

The reason I can relax, make the most of my freedoms and trust that there will always be work round the corner is that I have perspective. I have experienced the worst times, when there's no money to pay the mortgage and no one is replying to my emails. And, somehow, I have got through them. I have experienced the good times, when the phone won't stop ringing and you say 'Yes' to so many things that you wind up burning out completely. I know neither of these states last for ever. And I know I am still standing when they eventually end, having always learned something valuable from the experience.

These days, I realise that quiet times can be spent either worrying at home, staring at a computer screen and catastrophising about the future. Or they can be spent enjoying life, spending time with people we love and generally absorbing the absolute fucking brilliance of the world around us. It's not just what makes life worth living, it's what fuels the ideas that eventually pay the bills.

When I emerged from the Covid lockdown, I decided that I wanted to find a way of working from home full-time. Work is stressful but being close to my family was the best antidote. I had one of those garden offices built out the back of my house. It was small, warm and soundproof – and I hoped it would allow me to earn some sort of crust for the rest of my working days without ever having to stray far from home.

There are people who claim that we humans are naturally gregarious creatures who require interaction almost as urgently as food and water. I'm not convinced by that at all. I like the idea of being able to earn a living all alone in the confines of my glorified shed. I don't want face-to-face meetings. I don't need watercooler chit-chat. I will be delighted if I never have to sing 'Happy Birthday' to a vague acquaintance from bought ledger ever again. Sometimes, I find myself fantasising about retirement. To me, the garden office provides a stepping stone that I will have to make do with until (a) I win the lottery or (b) we finally reconstruct capitalism to allow us humans more time off to just play *FIFA* and listen to records.

In his brilliant book *Recovery: The Lost Art of Convalescence*, Dr Gavin Francis explains the magical healing benefits of rest, reflection, leisure and travel. In twenty years as a GP he has often found lifestyle changes like these to be more effective than any pharmaceutical prescription in helping patients regain and sustain good health. Which is obviously easier said than done in the ludicrously graft-centric society we live in today. As Dr Francis puts it: 'Self-compassion is a much-underrated virtue, and the rhythms of modern life are often antithetical to those of recovery.'

But why should we only focus on self-compassion when we are in a state of recovery from illness or trauma? A better idea is to try and practise this stuff, as much as possible, before we get sick in the first place. I'd like today's kids to grow up understanding that taking a bit of time out to do something you enjoy, getting some rest or just staring blankly out of the window for a half an hour every day is a worthwhile and important use of their time.

Unfortunately for my own kids, they will have to work for a living on account of me having no financial legacy to speak of. There will be nothing left for them once I'm gone. I'll probably have to flog the house at some point to pay for care so my children will be truly high and dry. Oh well; it might do them good, I suppose.

As long as they always understand, even if it's semi-secretly, inside their minds, that work is mostly a load of daft bollocks you have to do to survive. For most people it is an exploitative – almost perverse – power game in which an unscrupulous employer forces you to travel in and out of a depressing corporate headquarters every day on an overcrowded train in return for a piss-take of a wage. Most of us have no choice but to enlist – the trick is to not get brainwashed into thinking any of it matters beyond the cold, transactional process. One of my worst fears is that my children become the sort of people you sit next to at a work event who seem to take pleasure in talking about marketing strategy and unironically refer to the seasons of the year as 'Q1', 'Q2', 'Q3' or 'Q4' as if they're fucking C-3PO.

The fact that any of us still have to put in forty-hour weeks in this day and age is a scam dreamed up by the establishment to keep us exhausted and docile. Bertrand Russell (as quoted by Dr Francis in the book) was onto this years ago when he wrote:

> Modern methods of production have given us the possibility of ease and security for all; we have chosen instead to have overwork for some and starvation for others. Hitherto we have continued to be as energetic as we were before there were machines. In this we have been foolish, but there is no reason to go on being foolish forever.

He wasn't wrong, either. And bear in mind, he wrote that years before the emergence of AI and smartphones. Don't get me wrong, I enjoy what I do for a living. Even the process of writing this book is quite nice. But there must be an app out there that could do it just as well – if not better – while I lived off a universal basic income that could be funded by a tax on robots. If we were foolish back in 1935 when Russell penned *In Praise of Idleness*, we must be positively barmy to still be flogging our guts out in the 2020s.

I went up to the storage unit. It's always an emotional experience. In the dark and eerie basement of Big Yellow, Richmond, sits a five-foot-by-five-foot unit containing the relics, artefacts and assorted ephemera of my strange, scattergun career in the British media.

Hundreds of old magazines that I either wrote for or edited. Do I still really need that 1997 copy of *Men's Health* containing my 750 words on fitness classes for men? It was my first published piece in a proper mag. Or my cover story for the *NME* in 2007, when I went to New York to interview Scissor Sisters? Or that 2010 issue of *Heat* with Posh Spice on the cover under the headline I CAN'T GO ON! That shifted half a million copies and earned me a tidy bonus which paid for a nice holiday in Italy. Those columns from the *Guardian*, *Cosmo*, *Shortlist* and the Ryanair inflight magazine. Does the world really need these to be carefully archived? Do I?

So many memories swirl out of that storage unit whenever I unlock the padlock and swing open the door. It's like the bit in Indiana Jones when he opens the Ark of the Covenant. Only instead of ghosts and Nazis, I am haunted by old lads'-mag covers featuring Abi

Titmuss and long-forgotten interviews with Black Rebel Motorcycle Club.

But, ultimately, who gives a fuck? Not my kids, that's for sure. I tried to engage them in a chat about my archive but they were pretty cruel, casting doubt on my claims to have ever been a proper journalist. Now all they see me doing is going into the garden shed to record endless podcasts. Understandably, they don't regard this as a proper job. I tell them it puts food on the table. They roll their eyes at me.

There are dozens of micro-cassettes in the storage unit too, containing interviews with everyone from Tony Benn to Ridley Scott to Jimmy Savile to Brett Easton Ellis. Maybe I will get them digitised so I can listen back or put them out as pods. But what's the point? And the old showreels from my TV days, featuring me with a fine head of hair delivering facetious pieces to camera on the BBC and Channel 4. My son at least showed some interest in the video games show I used to present for a long defunct digital channel. He wanted to know if I ever received free games. I told him I did. But I didn't really. I was just trying to impress him.

I looked upon the boxes and boxes of my words – captured in print, video and audio form – and realised that it was costing me two hundred quid a month to keep them there, gathering dust. Why? So I could one day look back at all that bollocks and feel what, exactly? Proud? Nostalgic? I'm not really sure. I just feel annoyed to be honest.

So I rented a van and moved it all out. Some of it will be kept in my loft. But most of it will be pulped, shredded, recycled and turned into toilet rolls. I've found a company that will do it all for me for fifty-five quid plus VAT. That's how much it will cost me to destroy almost every tangible record of my twenty-eight years in the media.

Who gives a fuck? The best bits are upstairs in my head anyway.

Chapter 7

Stop Shitting Yourself
About Being Lazy

The 2011 film *Limitless*, starring Bradley Cooper and Robert De Niro, has got a lot to answer for.

Cooper plays a loser who sits around in his pants eating cereal all day, struggling to get started as a writer and lamenting the loss of his girlfriend, who ups sticks and leaves when his bullshit gets too much to take.

Then, one day, he is given a magic tablet that immediately switches on the large parts of his brain that have been lying dormant all his life, lending him laser focus, boundless energy, stunning emotional intelligence and razor-sharp analytical abilities. Overnight, he becomes creatively productive and physically dynamic. Within weeks he is professionally successful, rich, popular and attractive. The definitive scene, for me, features a suddenly lean and muscular Cooper running beside the Hudson River in New York while miraculously absorbing a teach-yourself-Japanese audiobook through his headphones.

Like pretty much every bloke I know who saw this film when it first came out, I was smitten by the idea that such a personal transformation might be possible. I chose to ignore the fact that the central plot device was an imaginary pill that did all the hard work for you. I told myself that, with just a little extra effort and determination, I too could learn Japanese, write a bestselling novel, run a three-minute mile and pay off my mortgage. I didn't have access to a magic pill but I did know a number of cocaine dealers, which I felt was the next best thing. Coke drove my energy and, for a short while, sparked my creativity somewhat. But the benefits were short-lived; quite quickly it all backfired into misery, fear, panic and the almost complete disintegration of a life that was perfectly OK in the first place.

It took the experience of addiction and recovery to wake me up to how futile the pursuit of the *Limitless* lifestyle was. Over years of sobriety, therapy and self-reflection I came to realise that life is not a competition to be the best at everything. Rather, it is about the pursuit of contentment as you define it.

Why had I allowed a Hollywood movie to define my goals? Why did I want to be richer, faster, more popular and better at Japanese than everyone else I knew? Probably because I had not thought clearly enough about the things that really made me happy and worked out how to pursue them effectively. It's much easier, when you're young especially, to refer to prefabricated templates for success and happiness. Too often, the most compelling templates are presented by master storytellers in the movie or TV industries.

I keep reading about the concept of 'Monk Mode', whereby you disappear completely for a period of time, cutting out both real life and online socialising in order to invest your attention into a specific area of self-improvement. Switch off your phone, disconnect your devices, stop shaving and just stay indoors reading books about investment strategies or core strength exercises for a month. Sounds fucking thrilling.

I don't understand why periods of quiet isolation need to be about anything more than relaxing. The very act of relaxing is self-improving in itself. There doesn't need to be a specific goal. Productivity needn't be your aim. Quite the opposite: short periods in which you do absolutely fuck all, allowing yourself to drift aimlessly without any specific purpose or endgame, allow your body and mind to rest and regenerate. Often, without even trying, I come up with some of my best ideas during periods of wanton indolence. The mind meanders about in a state of daydream, untethered by tedious processes or objectives. It recuperates from the dreary and exhausting business of active thought. And, eventually, it starts to playfully throw about unusual and entertaining ideas that it's usually too constricted to contemplate.

But other times it doesn't. It just sits there doing nothing, while I stare at the ceiling. And that's OK too. In fact, it is a vital part of staying healthy. You don't want to let it get out of hand. But setting the odd hour or two aside for a lovely bit of laziness is as important as remembering to floss your teeth, exercise or read. We are not robots and life is not a race.

There is shame associated with slothfulness. One man's monk mode is another's 'Goblin Mode'. Goblin mode also involves consciously withdrawing from circulation for a set period, only the aim is to reject personal dignity. It involves wearing onesies all day, eating nothing but Pringles, watching reality TV and so on. I get the vibe – that goblin mode's proponents are celebrating slobishness in an ironic way. But doing nothing needn't be about being slobbish. And you don't need to hide behind irony to justify it to yourself either. You don't need to wear Primark pyjamas or eat cholesterol-rich foods; neither do you need a scented candle or a cashmere blanket (like the Danish do, with their slightly smug version of goblin mode, called *hygge*). You don't need to learn anything or come out on the other side with a new life skill. Not everything needs to be about tangible achievement.

You don't need to be a monk, a goblin or a smug Dane. Sometimes, you can just sit on your arse, switch off and let your goal be nothing more (or less) than simple, beautiful, life-enriching rest.

I read that the prime minister of New Zealand, Jacinda Ardern, had quit her job suddenly. She had been just thirty-seven when she first won in 2017 and secured a second victory in 2020 with a landslide. At the start of 2023, months before the next election was due, at a time when most leaders would be gearing up to maintain their grasp on power with every fingernail, she exited the political stage. It made me feel so happy. What a beautiful thing to do and what a great example to everyone else in the world who is sticking around in a job that they are too exhausted to do properly.

I found her words on the subject very powerful:

> I'm leaving, because with such a privileged role comes responsibility – the responsibility to know when you are the right person to lead and also when you are not. I know what this job takes. And I know that I no longer have enough in the tank to do it justice. It's that simple. I am human, politicians are human. We give all that we can for as long as we can. And then it's time. And for me, it's time.

There is something so dignified about quitting when you're at the top.

I was also moved by the resignation of Jürgen Klopp as manager of Liverpool FC. I felt as if he quit in exactly the right way. Not because he needed 'a fresh challenge'. Not because he had 'taken the club as far as it can go'. Not because 'the project had reached a natural conclusion'. But because he was knackered and just needed a break. Or, as he put it: 'I am running out of energy...I cannot do it again and again and again.'

Klopp always had the bollocks to swerve the tedious, increasingly corporate-sounding language of the footballing world. People often exaggerated just how witty or 'left field' the German was. The truth is that he was just more willing than most to speak plainly about his feelings, responding to questions in a pretty straightforward and honest way, without fear of being exposed as a normal human being. Sometimes he lost his temper. Sometimes he responded to opaque journalistic questions by saying, 'Sorry, I don't understand.'

This, in a world as riddled with cliché, claptrap and platitudes as football, made him stand out as some sort of maverick firebrand. In normal life, I think Klopp would just come across as what he is: a pretty intelligent, averagely amusing, very decent, occasionally grumpy bloke. I think we'd all be more than happy to be regarded that way.

The example he set by being honest about his departure was extremely powerful. Kids look up to their footballing heroes and buy into the bullshit they ordinarily spout about 'giving 110 per cent' or feeling 'devoted to a club' or its fanbase.

It fuels the dangerous narrative that conformity, consistency, hard work, devotion to a cause and relentless goal setting is the only way to succeed in life. But that, of course, is a conspiracy designed to keep us grinding away at the levers of capitalism. Really, life is much better when you can find work you enjoy, treat it as lightly as possible and then jack it all in when it starts to get boring. If you can't jack it in (most of us can't) then it's always good to keep a healthy mental detachment from your job. You are not your work. Your own welfare needs to come first sometimes.

You should never give 100 per cent (let alone 110 per cent) of yourself to anything. Life is complicated and beautiful and to navigate your way through it without burning out completely you need to balance your time and energy carefully. The perfectionist narrative about throwing all your focus into the pursuit of singular dreams is irresponsible, unrealistic, ludicrously macho and totally impractical. There are strong fascistic vibes about the whole thing. As for all this 'I love the club and am committed to the fans' bollocks: it's just a childish game invented by daft-headed supporters who require other adults to offer them a sense of comfort.

I'm a West Ham fan. I don't need the West Ham manager to tell me via the media how much he appreciates my support and loves the club. I'm a fucking adult. I just want to watch us win and he's got a living to earn. We both have similar agendas; that's enough for me.

Fine, as a football manager you can have an affection for the fans. But you are an individual with your own life to lead. You have a family of your own. You can't let your life be run by a bunch of drunken strangers in replica shirts shouting your name from the stands. All of us must make decisions for ourselves. If we are too preoccupied with performative 'loyalty' to others and 'passion' for abstract notions, then we will neglect ourselves and our health will suffer.

Klopp knew this and that is why he had the balls not to sugar-coat his announcement. He just admitted the truth: he wanted to have a bit of a rest then maybe do something else.

What a lovely thing to say.

This is why I never bother making up excuses when refusing social invitations. I just say: 'Sorry, I can't come because I don't really want to.' That should be enough for any reasonable person to understand (although it might also explain why I rarely get invited to anything these days).

All of this suggests that success must always come at the expense of our other, more fundamental human needs, such as balance and comfort, curiosity and joy, rest and silence. We are raised in a culture that discourages the pursuit of these things. They are often stigmatised as signs of weakness, weirdness, self-indulgence or indolence. But they aren't: they are essential parts of our lives. If we go without them we get sick in the head and the body. What's more, we just waste our lives on pursuing barmy ambitions that knacker us out and yet, somehow, still leave us feeling unfulfilled. A bit like eating a Chinese meal.

It's fine to be ambitious, I guess. But it should only go so far. Klopp has won plenty of trophies with Liverpool. He's right not to make the mistake of those other Premier League grandees who just couldn't quit even after they'd won almost everything there was to win. Clinging to power is embarrassing and a bit grubby. Most leaders stay well past their sell-by date, driven to desperation – mostly by their egos. You see it in politics and football management all the time (Arsène Wenger being the absolute classic of the genre).

But it happens in all lines of work. Often, it's the result of people being institutionalised. They have done the same thing for so long they just can't imagine what a different life might look like.

It's scary moving on. But it's doable. It's rare you ever hear someone expressing regrets about quitting a job. But you hear people moaning about their current jobs every day. Personally, I've never stuck around in a job long enough to get too emotionally attached to it, much less institutionalised by it. I move on quickly. It's about self-care. My mum used to always say to me – about school, work or anything else that was getting me down and making me feel trapped – 'Sam, it's not a life sentence. Nothing is. Not even life sentences these days! They all get let out early for good fucking behaviour!'

Notwithstanding her slightly draconian attitude to criminal justice, my mum was right. By constantly reminding me that life was fluid and there were almost always other options, she instilled in me a sense of freedom. It's really important to perceive yourself as free. The moment you start to see yourself out of alternative options, life – particularly working life – can start to seem pretty suffocating.

I always have a plan B, C and D in my back pocket. Why? Because I feel as if I am protecting myself from exploitation by unscrupulous/annoying/useless employers and colleagues. Not to come over all Karl Marx or anything, but in all jobs someone will at some stage try to exploit you. The signs are subtle. The threats are never explicit. But in silent, nuanced ways we are reminded that the Sword of Damocles hangs above us constantly. The message is always something along the lines of, 'If you don't bend to my will you will put your job, your livelihood and the welfare of your children in peril.'

If life outside of your job feels like a terrifying vortex of despair then you will find yourself bending over backwards for your employer. This is why people work such long hours, do stuff that doesn't quite fit in with their own personal values, punch downwards, put up with wankers and feel obliged to answer emails at 10 p.m. on a Sunday. Fuck that. Fuck all of it.

Yes, not everyone can sit in their garden shed podcasting and writing bullshit for a living like I do. But you have to understand, I built a career out of making my own content specifically because I never wanted to have a boss ever again.

It was my top priority. I used everything I had learned over the course of my career, working with and for numerous other people, to fashion a lifestyle whereby I answered to pretty much no one and got to say and write whatever I wanted. I am aware not everyone can do this. I am not putting it forward as a universally feasible lifestyle choice. And I'm not about to start trying to flog my 'freedom system' as an overpriced and slightly implausible online course. I'm just telling you that I don't much like being told where to be, what to do and what time I need to turn up to do it. So I worked hard to find a way around all of that bollocks. Along the way, as I was accumulating all the experience I needed to get to this point, I accepted numerous jobs and quit almost all of them.

I wanted to keep seeking new working experiences. And I didn't want to hang around long enough for anyone to get sick of me. Most of all, I just wanted to feel free and in charge of my own destiny. Especially when I started a family. I just didn't want to feel as if my kids' future was somehow in the hands of some know-nothing in middle management. So I quit, I quit and I quit again. By God, it felt good.

Sometimes I didn't need to quit because the company I was working for just collapsed (I've been involved in a lot of start-ups and launches – they are exciting but terrifying). And once or twice I just didn't get my contract renewed, which is a bit like being sacked but not quite as humiliating. But mostly I quit. I always knew when the time was right. It was when I felt as if I was losing control of the stuff that made me happy or sad. If work was making me miserable and I was unable to make the changes necessary to improve the situation, I would just walk away. When I look back on my twenty-seven years of working, I can't think of a walkout that I regret.

Once I quit a job at a magazine because a management figure told me off for organising Christmas drinks without telling her about it first. I found this cheap, childish and absurd. I might have pitied her for being so small-minded had I not realised that she had some agency over me. The short, ugly exchange we shared in a cold meeting room neatly encapsulated the issues I'd had with the job for several months. I had found myself being engulfed in a relentless series of silly, playground-level disputes and petty political wrangles engineered by people I suspected were engaged in meaningless power games. It just made me unhappy and there wasn't enough good stuff to compensate for all the rubbish. So I quit without a second thought. Mind you, I can't say the company put up the biggest fight to keep hold of me. I got the impression that the final outcome was one that suited both parties. I was happy about that. They probably deserved someone who was more enthusiastic and less irritable than me, anyway.

When I look back on moments like that, I am proud that I always put myself as a human first and a working stiff second. I might not have realised it at the time, but I was always making professional decisions on the basis of my mental health. The only times my mental health suffered was when I didn't quit soon enough.

I would like to stress that you should be extremely fucking cautious about following any of my advice. This book is not meant to be a guide. I like to share my own thoughts and experiences in case they help the odd person relate and feel less alone. I am an imperfect case study and a deeply flawed tutor.

That said: if in doubt, fucking quit. You'll never look back.

* * *

A report in early 2024 claimed that Britain had one of the lowest productivity rates in the western world. That means we as a nation create less wealth per person than other, more conformist, societies such as France, Germany and the US. It's embarrassing, yes. But I also feel a bit proud.

It seems we put the hours in at work but don't really do much with them. I worked too hard in my twenties and thirties. Yes, I landed exciting jobs that were great fun and paid good money. Was that all down to talent and hard work? No, some of it was luck. Yes, hard work can often put you in the best position to catch a break. Most of us need to work hard to fulfil our ambitions. But I also know that I often just found myself in the right place at the right time. I was lucky in a ton of ways – not least the fact that I happened to be born and bred in London, which allowed me to get a foot in the door at the sort of media companies I wanted to work at while living at home, rent-free, with my mum. My mum worked much harder than me her whole life – as a secretary mostly – but never had the same luck. It's an insult to people like her to suggest that 'hard work' is all it takes to succeed. It's far more complex than that.

I'm sure there were a ton of people far more talented and worthy than me living in other parts of the country who just couldn't have found a practical way of doing six months on next to no wages in a magazine office in central London. Had they been able to do so, they might have had all the opportunities I had. We can all work hard but, more often than not, you also need a huge amount of luck and privilege to succeed. Those who tell themselves otherwise are deluded egotists living in their own juvenile hero fantasy.

Working hard is admirable. But not if you let it take priority over your wellbeing and happiness, on the promise that the graft will eventually make all your dreams come true. The Protestant work ethic, which hoodwinks its followers into thinking that God himself is keeping an eye on our clocking-in habits, is a ruse designed by the crafty bosses of yesteryear who gaslit peasants into helping them get rich. There used to be a legitimate quid pro quo at least. Now there are fewer guarantees of reward. You need to slack off for your own sanity sometimes, however unnatural that feels; you'll live longer and be happier.

Learning to like yourself is the best antidote to workaholism. It stops you from feeling bad about enjoying life. It stops you giving away your time and energy just to help others make money. Best of all, it allows you to take regular daytime naps without feeling an ounce of guilt. Try it.

I was finally struck down with Covid on the day I turned forty-eight. This was 2023, long after the virus was trendy. It was just like when I bought a NutriBullet in 2017 and all the millennials I was working with at the time teased me for being late to the party. I couldn't stop going on about juicing but nobody wanted to listen because, as a conversation topic, it felt old, stale and tedious.

By the spring of 2023, nobody was taking Covid very seriously any more. There were vaccines and there was know-how too. The sense of panic and alarm the word 'Covid' once generated was already a distant memory for most people. I'd had three jabs so I figured I was either never going to get it or the symptoms would be imperceptible. But I was wrong.

On my very special day, as I sat watching football on the telly with a nice big slice of the birthday cake that my mum had just dropped round, I was suddenly struck by a sense of dizziness. Next, my limbs started to ache and my body started to shiver with cold. I staggered upstairs to my bed and covered myself in three blankets. Still the shivering didn't stop. I had to stick on the electric blanket for the first time since February. Eventually, I drifted into a troubled sleep.

When I woke up, two hours later, I was drenched in sweat, kicking the blankets off myself and scrambling for water. It was immediately clear: after three years of acting smug because I had managed to swerve the virus, it had now come to get me when I was least expecting it. And it had got me bad.

I spent ten days in bed, quarantined, away from my family, too feeble to get off my arse, barely able to read a book or even think straight. My head felt like it was full of Ready Brek. Even a short walk to the bathroom necessitated a three-hour recovery. At night I was unable to sleep at all. My mind came alive with anxiety at about two in the morning and I just had to lie, staring into the darkness, turning over a series of worst-case scenarios.

After day three or four I started to lean into the whole thing a bit more. I realised that, ordinarily, I felt physically healthy but mentally on edge due, in no small part, to the constant sensory stimulation of modern life and the nagging sense that I should be getting more done. These are the twin curses of being human in the twenty-first century. Everything is so non-stop. The only sustained respite I can remember came during the initial few months of lockdown back in 2020. While it was horrific for many, I was lucky enough to enjoy a fleeting moment in which the world seemed to stop turning and all the feelings of guilt, suffocation, fear and self-loathing were replaced by a certain peace.

Three years later, in my isolation, I was feeling something similar. Lying in my pit, physically derelict, I at least felt mentally and emotionally calm. I was unable to work. I was barely able to communicate. Who cared? It was nice to just stop giving a shit about things for a while. No deadlines, no pitches, no catch-ups, no meetings. I wrestled myself up once every couple of days to send out emails cancelling things with messages that barely bothered with courtesy. 'Sorry, I have to reschedule, I have Covid.' Jesus, it felt good.

Admittedly, announcing you have Covid didn't elicit the same sort of sympathy it once did. People just didn't buy the fact that this virus could still kick your head in, even if you're vaccinated and relatively healthy like me. They respond with a bit of scepticism, as if I was claiming to have an illness that no longer existed or was not nearly bad enough to justify skipping stuff or cancelling work. But I didn't care what they thought. I felt so ill that other people's perceptions no longer mattered. I had been set free by sickness.

I managed to glance at social media once a day and noticed that people were still taking the time and energy to shout bullshit at each other about matters they could not control. I smiled to myself as I watched them scrap and debase themselves for attention. And I felt as if I was floating above all the madness. Happy to be irrelevant and content with my incapacity. Covid is hell, yes. But it ain't half emancipating.

Chapter 8

Stop Shitting Yourself
About Having Fun

Luke Ambler is a former rugby league pro from Halifax who founded the extraordinary support group Andy's Man Club. It's a national network of weekly get-togethers where blokes get to share a cup of tea and a chat about what's going on in their lives. I attended one in Peterborough in 2018 and was taken aback by how easy it was to settle into an open, honest and friendly conversation with a bunch of strangers.

People are always on about how important it is for men to talk about their feelings, but until that day I never quite understood why. The atmosphere in the room was really relaxed, warm and down to earth. It didn't feel remotely new age, woo-woo, earnest or patronising. Until then, I'd strongly suspected that all formalised attempts to get men to be vulnerable would be all those things. But Andy's Man Club was bullshit-free, sometimes fun and rooted in the idea that our problems are easier to cope with once we realise we are not alone.

As I keep saying, one of the hardest parts of being a man is the pathological competitiveness. We can compete to be the strongest and most together in the room. Entering a room filled with people who are specifically there to drop the bullshit and admit to the fact that they're struggling – sometimes with big stuff, often the little things – is so liberating. You open your mouth, talk a bit about the stuff that's making you feel crap that week and by doing so you feel stronger. Admitting your struggles makes you feel grown up and confident. Posturing like your life is perfect suddenly seems like embarrassing playground stuff by comparison.

Anyway, I interviewed Luke Ambler for the newspaper a few weeks later because I had been so impressed by his group. He set it up in the aftermath of the suicide of his brother-in-law, Andy. Andy had been a personable and upbeat bloke who had shown no signs of wanting to take his own life. Ambler was convinced that, had he felt able to open up and admit his feelings without fear of ridicule or shame, Andy would still be alive. And so he started the club in his memory, with the intention of halving the male suicide rate in the UK. Thousands of men now attend the meetings up and down the country every Monday night at 7 p.m. It's a beautiful thing.

When I met with Luke, he embodied the way he had managed to create an organisation that appealed to just the sort of ordinary blokes who might usually have felt sceptical about mental health, group therapy and all that stuff. Luke is six-foot-four with a broad Yorkshire accent; down to earth, funny and relaxed. He was not like the weird school counsellor in sandals. He was the exact opposite. It was disarming.

During our chat, in a busy cafe at King's Cross station, a waiter walked past our table and knocked a drink over. Water splashed everywhere, over the table surface, into our laps and onto the floor. It was a brief moment of chaos that threatened to send me into a micro-panic. But Luke, without missing a beat, stood up immediately, grabbed a roll of kitchen paper from the counter, ripped off a huge wad and soaked up the mess in a few seconds, while continuing to answer my question. It was all over in the blink of an eye. He had sorted it out without fussing, worrying, getting annoyed or complaining. It was just a tiny moment but it made a lasting impact: as someone who can find himself flying off the handle in response to the most trivial of problems, I was bowled over by the no-nonsense, completely unemotional reaction that Luke displayed.

Life can seem so complicated sometimes. Often it's just a pile-up of little irritants that can send you into a spiral: an unexpected bill arrives, your internet stops working, you can't find anywhere to park, the tap in the bathroom won't stop dripping. Whatever. When I'm tired and haven't been keeping an eye on myself, these small problems feel like massive challenges that sometimes make me stressed, sometimes make me angry and often just make me a bit sad. I try to look at the way that more calm and relaxed men live their lives. Not the ones who say you have to push yourself to the limit to be happy and successful. But people like Luke who prefer to keep things simple. Who don't fool themselves into thinking that they can somehow insulate themselves from life's problems. But who, instead, resolve to take those problems in their stride with an unemotional, calm and practical approach.

I enjoy the company of men who have made their own decisions about their identity and lifestyle and don't bother themselves worrying about what other people think. I aspire to be like them. Sometimes I manage it. But in the meantime I just try to take inspiration from the handful of unique blokes who seem to have cracked it.

Not all of them are as down to earth as Luke Ambler, mind you.

Once upon a time, when I was a magazine editor, I received an email written entirely in caps. I used to get tons of emails every day back then and tended to ignore 90 per cent of them. But I've always understood that anyone who writes exclusively in capital letters is worth paying attention to, either because they are important, angry, mad or all three. This particular email was from the filmmaker, restaurant critic and bon viveur Michael Winner – a man I had always found fascinating but had never had any personal dealings with. He had a new book out and wondered if I would like to collect my copy in person FROM HIS HOUSE! I was so excited that I whizzed over to his impressive pile in Kensington almost immediately.

I don't know what I was expecting to get out of my visit, beyond a free book that I was unlikely to actually ever read. Maybe just a selfie, a snoop around the house and a couple of anecdotes about the making of his movie *Death Wish*. That would have been enough for me. But, as it transpired, the afternoon I spent with this (now departed) show-biz raconteur provided me with some of the wisest, most inspirational, educational, unusual and entertaining pieces of life advice I ever received. Rarely a day goes by without me thinking about the stuff Winner told me on that sunny afternoon in 2010.

He was charm personified. We went down to the cinema in his basement where he had prepared a gift bag for me, containing a nice bottle of champagne and some signed copies of his books. We talked down there most of the afternoon. He had some forthright views on restaurant service, as you might expect, and a bunch of celebrity tales. But I found the details of his lifestyle more fascinating than anything else. He told me that he drove everywhere in London, avoiding traffic by using the bus lanes. 'The cameras hardly ever catch you so I might get two three-hundred-pound fines a year, which works out quite cost effective,' he said. He would park directly outside whichever restaurant he was visiting, leaving the motor on a yellow line while he ate. He reasoned that the parking ticket was only sixty pounds – the same price as a return taxi fare. 'And the difference is I don't have to walk around in the rain looking for taxis. I just leave the restaurant and step straight back into my car.' There was a certain logic to his extravagance that I found very convincing.

He was upset that a newspaper had recently run a story claiming that he stole sweets from his local cinema. 'Someone took a picture of me helping myself to the pick-and-mix then jumping the queue for a movie,' he lamented. 'What they don't know is that I pay the manager of that cinema one thousand pounds a month in order to do that whenever I please. So it's not theft at all. In fact, seeing as I only visit the place once in a while, they're making a very healthy profit from the arrangement!'

He was more quietly spoken and humble than his public persona might indicate. He suggested that the whole cigar-chomping, posh-dickhead thing was just a daft routine. I wound up believing him. 'I'm not very sociable at all,' he said. 'Most nights I have an early dinner, then go upstairs and watch a movie in bed. I only go out to eat about once a week.' With whom? I asked. 'Michael Caine usually,' he shrugged.

Next we went up to the bedroom. It was the size of a football pitch, with a gargantuan bed sitting in the middle on a raised platform. The huge windows looked out over spectacularly beautiful gardens. He waved at his neighbour in the adjacent garden. 'Isn't that Jimmy Page?' I asked, making out the figure of the Led Zeppelin guitarist.

'Yes, it is.' He beamed.

The films Michael Winner made weren't all that great, were they? But he wouldn't tell you any different. He didn't seem to regard himself as anything special and saw the world he lived in as completely absurd.

He gave me one last piece of advice as I left. 'Don't take this the wrong way, but you see that bit of hair that's receding at the front of your head?' I touched my wispy fringe self-consciously and nodded. 'You should wash that in lager. It helps it grow back. But I only use Heineken, the rest doesn't work so well.'

I tried it the next day. It didn't work. He'd been taking the piss out of me just like he continually took the piss out of himself. But most of all he took the piss out of life – just like all of us dream of doing. Not many have the wit or the balls to do it with quite the same panache as Winner.

There's a great deal to hate about football these days. The dirty money, the flagrant corruption, the aggressive promotion of gambling companies that facilitate addiction and suicide. And then there are the persistent elements of racism, homophobia and whatever other ugly intolerances coked-up fans can conjure and chant about. Urgh. What a cesspit the beautiful game has become. And yet I just can't quit my football habit. A man like me has nowhere else to go. I love watching football, playing football, talking, thinking and dreaming about football and I won't ever be able to stop. I like it because it is simple and exciting and, yes, sometimes beautiful. But more than the stuff on the pitch, I love what football has given me personally: a lifetime of memories and experiences that would not otherwise have existed but for my hopeless, romantic devotion to what is, essentially, a daft children's game.

More than anything, football gave me friendship. Growing up in west London while supporting West Ham, a team from the other side of the city, wasn't easy. There were Chelsea and QPR fans. There were even a few who followed Spurs and Liverpool. But supporting an unsuccessful club that lived twenty-six stops away on the District Line just provoked playground bemusement and ridicule. So when I met another kid cursed with the same strange West Ham fixation as me, the bond we formed was instant and long-lasting. We shared a niche worldview and set of formative experiences that few others could ever understand. This is how I met my best mate Ollie, when I was six, both wearing West Ham shirts on a school trip to a canal in Brentford. One spring week in 2022 the two of us, now both middle-aged, travelled to Spain to watch West Ham play Seville. We lost the game but the trip – thirty-six hours across Europe full of laughter and stupidity and nostalgia and a pervading sense of carefree optimism that is all too rare in middle age – was magical.

When we were away we learned that Roman Abramovich had been relieved of his ownership of Chelsea football club by the government as part of sanctions bought against oligarchs following Russia's invasion of Ukraine. Of course, there was a great deal of celebration and gloating among West Ham fans. But I wondered what would happen to those Chelsea fans Ollie and I once bickered with in the playground; they would be old like us now. Their friendships and memories and parts of their identity would be married to their club just like ours were; if the club somehow died so too would a part of them. I generally deplore the corny romanticism of the dewy-eyed football fan. I find the marketing that surrounds football fandom, focused as it usually is on a mixture of dreary bants and mawkish sentimentality, to be patronising and trite. That said, the existential crisis faced by Chelsea and, by extension, football in general, made me face the facts. Football really has played an important part in my life. I'm not particularly proud of that, but there we have it. It's just a game but it's a game that's capable of bringing people together in a meaningful way. It generates bonds, connections, humanity and joy. It's such a shame that we let a bunch of cynical bastards use their money to exploit all of that love. Sometimes I wish I'd just got into stamp collecting.

A year later, West Ham managed to reach the final of the UEFA Conference League. We would face the Italian team Fiorentina in Prague, Czech Republic. And I would be there with two of my oldest mates, Nev and Dan. We travelled across Europe together by train, plane, taxi and by foot. It was probably the most enjoyable few days of my entire life. West Ham won the cup and I was there to see them do it. My mates and I sang and danced and hugged, celebrating the sort of victory we had long since concluded was never going to be gifted to West Ham supporters like us. But we did it. And, I can tell you, it is the best feeling in the world.

Although emotions ran high and the atmosphere was heavily fuelled by copious amounts of Czech lager all round, the thought of me having a drink never crossed my mind. Why would it? I was experiencing unbelievable feelings of pure, distilled joy; the sort of joy I had been waiting for my whole life. Sporting victory, friendship, adventure, glory, sunshine and an overwhelming sense of connection with all the other Hammers around the world. This is the shit we live for. Why would I need to embellish that with alcohol? It would have just blurred the edges of those beautiful emotions. I didn't want to numb myself. I wanted to feel every last bit of it. And I did.

I'm so glad this victory arrived when I was sober. Because if it had happened in my drinking days I would have pissed the whole wonderful experience away by boozing myself into a state of oblivion.

When you're contemplating giving up the alcohol, you think everyone will turn it into a big deal. Especially if you're abstaining on a special occasion. But nobody gave a fuck that I wasn't drinking. Nobody noticed. Nobody asked. That's the thing: in truth, nobody is paying much attention to what you are or aren't drinking. When life gets as exciting as it had been over those past few days, people are just locked in the moment.

Most of the people around me were pissed. I was delighted for them. However, one of my mates was sober like me and we bumped into a few others who had chosen the same path as us. It didn't really make a difference to anyone. You could have easily mistaken the sober ones for being drunk anyway. When those feelings hit me, I don't need to consume a special drink to make me act barmy – I will do it anyway. We were there to have fun and feel love and that's what we all did, drunk or sober.

There were five thousand West Ham fans packed into the small stadium in Prague but at least another thirty thousand were spread all over the city; they had travelled without tickets just to be part of the event. It was incredible to be around so many other people who felt the same passion, love and excitement as I did. I kept seeing people I knew or had once known, like one of those weird dreams where random figures from your past and present all congregate in some random place.

Before the match there was nothing but excitement and enthusiasm; good will and joy spilled out of everyone as friends and strangers alike chatted, hugged, sang and shared in what was very close to being a spiritual experience. After the match it was like time stood still. All of us had become accustomed to a deep certainty that, however much we loved West Ham, however loyal we were to them, they would always, ultimately, let us down. But suddenly, here we all were, with our collective pessimism confounded, trying to process emotions that were as unfamiliar as they were unexpected.

I didn't quite know what to do with myself. At one point I took my top off. Later that night, I found myself in a disco dancing to Boney M.'s 'Daddy Cool', clutching a vegetarian sausage roll in one hand and a Heineken Zero in the other.

All sorts of other beautiful, strange, uplifting and wonderful little moments unfolded over the next couple of days. Long after the final whistle, my mates and I walked back to our Airbnb from the stadium, wandering through the dark, dramatic streets of the Czech capital, embracing every other Hammer we encountered along the way, reflecting on the moment we'd been waiting for all of our lives. Drinking it in.

Life is just a collection of moments. Treasure the magic ones. You don't have to honour them by getting off your tits. You can just live through them and relish every last drop of ecstasy they deliver.

Is it childish to be so emotionally invested in a children's game? Probably. But there is no rulebook on how you should draw pleasure from life.

And anyway, it wasn't just about the eleven men in claret and blue winning the football match. It was about the human connection I felt with the thousands of other West Ham fans who had shared the same feelings and experiences over so many decades and had been compensated for all that pain and anguish by just one glorious night in Prague.

I'd heard it said that the opposite of addiction is connection. That week in Prague, I discovered it to be true.

Not all moments of joy need to be packaged in foreign trips and magnificent sporting triumph. I am equally moved by the small, daily pleasures that permeate our lives for free. For me, music is the biggest and the best. When I moved into my neighbourhood fifteen years ago, I was aware that the local boozer had a small venue out the back that was somewhat renowned in jazz circles. But I was in my early thirties and thought jazz was daft and pretentious, for posturing weirdos and earnest chin-strokers in berets and polo necks. I was foolish and ignorant.

Things change. I started secretly listening to jazz a few years ago, strictly as an accompaniment to work. I found that the meandering, lyric-free sounds somehow aided my writing process. I kept the output of John Coltrane and Thelonious Monk contained on my AirPods, too ashamed to let the world know that I was 'using' jazz to drive my productivity. You must understand that, initially, I didn't like the music. I was abusing jazz. It helped focus my thoughts and navigate me gently into a state of work-hypnosis. There is probably some sort of neuro-scientific explanation for all this that I am too lazy to look up.

In lockdown, I bought a book of mid-century design that featured a number of beautiful covers for albums by the likes of Miles Davis, Stan Getz and Dave Brubeck. My father-in-law, a true and unashamed lifetime jazzer, caught wind of my interest in the aesthetics surrounding the music. Next thing I know, he'd sent me some records in the post. Entry-level stuff, really. Nothing too dangerous. But I began to play these discs occasionally, whenever I found myself alone in the house, while I sipped a coffee and stroked the cat. Soon, I realised I was starting to enjoy the way these strange noises were making me feel.

Cut to the autumn of 2022 and my mate Hack and I are squished into the tiny jazz club I once vowed never to attend. We are watching a band composed of men decades older than us, with grey hair, wrinkled skin and unfashionable trainers. They are performing with such skill, passion and enthusiasm that it is making us both feel quite emotional. By the end, the jazz has mutated into more of a groove. We are both up on our feet, dancing, shoulder to shoulder with the rag-tag audience of local old folk, curious out-of-towners on a pilgrimage and the dyed-in-the-wool jazz people who are here every night. Hack and I are among the youngest in the audience. What we love, perhaps even more than the music, is the lust for life, the unselfconscious glee and the unapologetic un-coolness of the people around us.

As middle age trundles on, and I start to see my autumn years on the distant horizon, I sometimes worry. What will life be like when my man boobs are sagging and my trainers are bought from the supermarket? Does the loss of edge have to mean the loss of purpose, fun and vitality? Or does it, in fact, mean the opposite? Could it be that the jazzers were right all along? That worrying less about how you look and more about how you feel represents true liberation.

A gig up the river at the O2 Arena by a 'legacy' band I used to watch on *Top of the Pops* in the nineties costs upwards of a hundred quid and is a right hassle to get to. The local jazz joint costs me a tenner, I can walk there and back in minutes, I hear music that I have never heard before played up close in a manner that is fascinating and nobody gives a shit when I get up and start dancing really badly. That's living all right. Turns out I wasn't too good for jazz – jazz was too good for me. But not any more.

I have also been to see a Smiths tribute band. They're called The Smyths. It was in a back room of a local pub and it was life affirming. It helped that I love the music of the actual Smiths. It also helped that the pretend Morrissey didn't come with the iffy political baggage and silly racism of the real Morrissey and I therefore didn't need to wrestle with any of my tedious liberal scruples over enjoying his performance. But most of all it was about the atmosphere in the room, as the sounds of rainy eighties Manchester whipped an audience of clapped-out, middle-aged bastards like me into an improbable state of ecstasy. The familiar bittersweet lyrics that narrated our youth laced with those euphoric melodies: it had a narcotic effect on the hundred or so parents (and maybe a few grandparents) who had walked through the doors moments earlier, worrying about whether their aching backs would be able to survive the evening. By the encore, there were men and women – who looked like they might not have cracked a smile since the mid-nineties – dancing, singing, hugging and even crying with joy. It was lovely. Strange where you can stumble upon spiritual experiences if you keep your eyes and mind open.

* * *

I found a new source of wellbeing from the seemingly small sense of satisfaction of doing puzzles. It's completely changed my outlook. Before, I'd never been much of a morning person. Through good times and bad, whether getting up in the dark to attend a job I hated or sleeping in late before a day of leisure, I'd always found the first few moments of the day really unpleasant. I'd wake up feeling scared. I'm never quite sure of what. If my mind is a filing cabinet, which I have to keep well organised, I feel as if vandals get in there at night, start opening all the drawers and throwing the important papers around. I wake up feeling discombobulated and unsure of my ability to confront the future. There could be some scientific explanation to do with cortisone levels, but what difference would it make to know? I'd been struggling like this every morning since childhood. I was past caring what the cause was; I just wanted a cure.

Since I got really, really into puzzles, I have started waking up feeling happy and optimistic. When I hear the alarm, I fling back the covers and stand upright almost immediately. I scuttle downstairs merrily to feed the pets and stick the kettle on. I open the blinds and smile into the sunlight. Sometimes, I even have a little whistle.

Concise crosswords were the gateway drug. My wife has been a big fan for years; I have always teased her for being a nerd. Crosswords seemed a bit too conventional and spoddy for me. I had an idea of myself as a renegade who lives too fast and burns too bright for the gentle pleasures of word-based conundrums. But, of course, the idea I have of myself is – and always has been – wrong. Like many washed-up, middle-aged men, I clung to a daft adolescent fantasy for a bit too long. The more I give into reality and accept that I am perhaps more Stephen Fry than Steven Tyler the more relaxed I seem to feel about life.

The thing that put me off crosswords for the first forty-eight years of my life was that I was shit at them. Insecure and weak-willed, I have always given up on stuff pretty quickly the moment I realise that I lack natural aptitude.

It's a shamefully late realisation, I know, but there is huge satisfaction in making gradual progress as a result of continued practice. Who knew? I do *The Times* crossword each day, painstakingly stumbling through each clue in order and then repeating until the whole thing is complete, or near enough. Once I'm done, I am overwhelmed by a sense of soft, warming self-satisfaction. It's a bit like the quiet smugness I feel after a morning run, only much less messy and undignified.

After a few weeks of crossword use, I started exploring other brainteasers: Wordle (you know, the game that was trendy about six years ago), connection puzzles, even a bit of Sudoku. I'm not exaggerating when I say they give me a thrilling little buzz. I think it must be the focus they demand; I've always enjoyed escaping into pastimes that block out all the other troubling thoughts and chaotic feelings that swirl around inside me. There was a time when booze and drugs provided the escape, but that proved to be unsustainable. Video games sometimes do the job, but slouching in front of the telly playing a football-management simulation doesn't do much for your self-respect when you're a forty-nine-year-old father of two with bills to pay and dinner to cook.

Puzzles, on the other hand, are meditative yet improving; a distraction that both numbs and nourishes. I am angry at myself for discovering their brilliance so late in life. I've spent thousands on therapy over the years. I'm not sure puzzling necessarily helps me unpick the great conundrum of my true identity and purpose in life, but it has helped me to relax and shown me that I am capable of progress through persistence.

These days, I don't wake up thinking, *SHIT SHIT SHIT! WHERE AM I?! WHAT'S HAPPENING?! WHY IS LIFE SO INTIMIDATING?* like I used to. Instead, the first thing I think is, *Seize the day! Grasp the nettle! It's time for another morning of puzzling!*

All of this has changed the focus of my work. I received an email from a stranger who said they enjoyed my writing 'despite the fact it was often depressing'. Wow. I had no idea. Certainly, when I was younger, most of the stuff I wrote was trying to be funny. Without noticing it, it seems I've tempered this somewhat as I've got older and drifted into misery memoir. Time was, I only wrote, spoke or behaved to elicit a few cheap laughs. Metaphorically (and sometimes literally) I spent the first few decades of my life pulling my pants down in the hope that passers-by would clap and cheer.

These days, I try to be a bit more honest about what is going on in my life and my head. Some people might find it all a bit downbeat. Certainly, a great deal of it is mundane. But the gentle ebbs and flows of my life, as I approach the tail end of my forties, offer me almost nothing but sweet, peaceful and unremarkable pleasures. I could write about sex, excitement, rock 'n' roll and all the other stuff we believe might deliver joy when we are younger. I mean, I'd have to reach pretty deep into my mental archives to accurately remember what most of those things felt like. But it wouldn't really be honest or authentic. It would give no indication of my actual experience of being alive and therefore nothing real or meaningful for anyone else to connect with.

Instead I write and talk about my love of jazz and puzzles, the losing battle I am fighting against my waistline or the fact that I went to see a Smiths tribute band in the local pub and really, really, really enjoyed it.

This is real life. It might not be blockbuster stuff but I love it. There is fun, absurdity and fulfilment in every last detail. There always has been but, when I was younger, I just couldn't see it. I was brainwashed by TV, glossy magazines and the influence of my equally naive peers into believing that life's only pleasures lay in high-speed glamour and excitement. In being the best. I devoted a huge amount of my energy into chasing that stuff only to find, once I'd had my fill, that it did nothing to enrich my worldview, nourish my soul or put a smile on my face. In fact, it often seemed to do the opposite of all those things.

There is nothing like getting to middle age and opening your heart to the wondrous beauty of the humdrum.

Revelling in domestic routine and the minutiae of bog-standard family life might once have looked to me like surrender. Now, I know it to be something far more profound: a realisation that all the contentment and joy I need is sitting right here in front of me. I used to think life could be so boring. Now I realise that I was just being unimaginative.

Chapter 9

Stop Shitting Yourself
About Calming the Fuck Down

My cat died on a stormy Sunday afternoon in October. His name was Nelson. He was pretty old and had lived a pretty full life, as far as cats' lives go. I bought him from a woman outside Hammersmith tube station for an extortionate £170. She turned up cupping the tiny creature in her hands, sodden with rain. I pushed the cash into her hand, snatched the cat and drove off home in my car where I presented him to my wife as a birthday gift. Nelson was frail and scared; the woman had assured me he was eight weeks old but the vet said he looked no more than a fortnight. Too young to be taken from his mother. It seemed unlikely he would survive.

But my wife and I nursed him diligently for those first few weeks and he fought through. I think that's why I formed such an extra special bond with him. He kinda thought I was his mum.

At the time, we had a couple of pretty tough Russian Blues living next door to us. They would jump over the fence to bully Nelson. Sometimes they would even enter our house through his cat flap and make themselves very much at home. He was terrified. To be honest, so was I. Their names were Oscar and Archie and they reminded me of the Kray twins. In the end, we had to move.

While the new house was being renovated, Nelson moved in with my mother-in-law. But she had a malicious Bengal called Hector living next door who was even more trouble than Oscar and Archie. Hector terrorised Nelson throughout his stay. It was a case of out of the frying pan and into the fire.

Finally, at the home we live in now, he settled. The local cats were generally respectful. They seemed to have a nice little feline community going, where bullying wasn't an issue. Nelson was happy and calm. But one day during lockdown the back door slammed shut in a sudden gust of wind and caught Nelson's tail. It was broken in two places. He had to be operated on twice. At one point it looked like he might have to face an amputation. They fixed him eventually but I'm not sure he ever 100 per cent recovered from the trauma.

Although this all sounds as if he had a life of unrelenting anxiety, there was always a lot of love around Nelson. He was an affectionate cat who was always right at the heart of everything the family did. He wasn't housebound – he liked going out to do cat stuff in the streets once in a while. But he would put his time in at home too, sitting on my lap while I watched Netflix, interfering with my laptop while I was trying to work, always trying to steal the poppadoms from our Friday-night curry order.

My favourite moments were when I would come in late from a night at the football and he would be waiting to greet me on the arm of the sofa. I'd stroke him for a while and chat to him quietly, telling him about my day. He'd stare into my eyes like he was really listening and purr enthusiastically. I found it very soothing. There was a reassuring permanence to him; a reliable calmness; a consistent warmth. He genuinely made me feel better when times were rough. He was my mate.

And then we came home from lunch at my mum's that Sunday and he was lying in one of his usual spots, quite peacefully. I knelt down to stroke him and realised he wasn't breathing. Strangely, when I realised he was dead, I felt a bit annoyed. *Why did you have to die, Nelson?* I thought. We adopted him just after our first kid was born, fifteen years ago. He'd been an integral part of the family unit ever since. Then he was gone and I was gutted. I sat with the feelings of pain. I didn't try to shy away or bury them. I knew that it might seem daft to an outsider, but I didn't care. This was a bit of raw pain that I wanted to experience. Because I wanted to honour him. This is the sort of emotion that for many years I hid from. I now realise that was a shame because sometimes you can't fully feel love without the pain that goes with it.

Anyway, a few weeks after he died, I bought a new kitten and called him Bobby. And shortly after that, a cockapoo we called Cookie arrived. And so begun the new era of faeces-strewn pandemonium.

It started on 27 December 2023, when the family hit the road to a breeder's farm in Norfolk where I handed over the price of a half-decent second-hand hatchback in return for this three-month-old cockapoo. Cookie was beautiful and cuddly but we couldn't help but notice in the car journey home that she stank. She stank of dog. Was it naive of us to imagine that our dog would be a special dog that smelled of peaches or lavender? Yes, it was. And our naivety didn't end there.

The thing about having a puppy is that you are constantly thinking about another creature's bowel movements. My days used to be quite relaxed and pleasant. A little gym session in the morning, a bit of writing in the afternoon, knock up a bowl of pasta for dinner, then watch the box until bedtime. Lovely. Now my schedule is entirely built around when Cookie might next need the toilet. I watch her constantly, trying to spot the signs of an impending poo or wee. I take her out in the garden at night and implore to do her business. She sniffs about and starts to play. I don't want her to play. It is cold and dark and I want her to just get it over with. Sometimes I use the torch on my phone to check what she is up to. Shining a light at a dog's bumhole at one in the morning is a sobering experience, I can tell you.

Of course, she is also destroying things. And she fights with the cat non-stop. The house is in a state of utter mayhem. I try to get her to sit peacefully with me in my office while I work. I have to try and generate some earnings between faeces-management sessions. But she whines and scratches at the office door.

Why did we get a dog? Maybe because so many of the men I have interviewed about their mental health on my podcast tell me that dog ownership has helped them profoundly. The positive reviews of canine husbandry were so overwhelmingly positive that I just had to try it. I had a dog when I was a kid that I really loved. But that was the eighties when you didn't have to walk them that much and, when you did, no one expected you to pick up their crap in little bags. It's a lot more work these days.

I envisaged my dog-owning life to be one of meditative walks in the park or life-affirming cuddles by the fire. But those things haven't quite materialised yet. There have been some pleasant strolls together and numerous cuddles (although these have been a bit more intense and licky than life affirming). But to be honest I just feel overwhelmed and exhausted. I feel daft admitting it because she's just a puppy. How hard can it be? Well, harder than I expected. I don't regret the decision, mind you. I know I sound like I do, but I really don't. Cookie is adorable. There is a real sense of love between all of us. I have faith that the teething problems will eventually smooth themselves out.

She will grow and mature and learn that iPhone cables are not food.

This experience has been another reminder that real life is more complex and challenging than the two-dimensional versions we are presented with on social media. I have posted a few pictures of Cookie looking gorgeous and docile on Instagram. I got a ton of likes. Puppies are super popular. But if I want to be of service to other prospective dog owners, perhaps I should post a few more of her shitting on the rug.

* * *

In the late seventies my parents took my three older brothers and me to north Wales for a fortnight. I've no idea why they identified this place as a holiday destination; I can't understand how anyone chose a holiday before the internet. Did we really just walk into a high-street travel agent and ask them what they had on offer? Seems a bit risky in retrospect, doesn't it? These days I like to check every review on Tripadvisor, every image on Google Earth and every video on YouTube before I even think about committing a deposit. In the seventies, you just got in your car, crossed your fingers and headed out on the motorway into the great unknown.

I was just a baby on this Wales trip. Apparently, I cried all the way there in the car and throughout most of the holiday. My brothers still seem pissed off about this whenever the subject comes up. I don't see what they expect to achieve by guilt-tripping me four decades years later.

What do they want from me? Financial compensation? Just move on, lads. Anyway, despite my crying, I'm told everyone else had a great time on that holiday. It gets talked about quite a lot, perhaps because it was the last time our family went away together and created what might have passed for golden memories before my parents split just a few months later.

Many times I have heard tell of that wondrous fortnight spent playing in rolling sand dunes and on sprawling, sandy beaches. I've heard about the walks through magical woodland, the waterfalls, the friendly people and the steam-train rides. I remember none of this, of course, but it's always lived as an idyllic fantasy in my imagination.

So, aged forty-eight, I decided to try and recreate it with my own little family. Obviously, I researched the shit out of the whole trip for months in advance before hitting the road in the last week of August. Still, I didn't quite know what to expect. My kids (then aged fifteen and ten) were clearly underwhelmed by the prospect of a summer holiday that didn't involve flying anywhere. So, I really needed north Wales to over-deliver.

The drive out of London, up through the Midlands and across the border into Wales was not immediately exhilarating. The kids sulked in the back with their headphones in. Then Snowdonia National Park emerged on the horizon and the sun crept through the clouds. Eventually, in the gaps between the mountains, we saw the coast. It was breathtaking. The sort of aesthetically enchanting arrival you just don't get from touching down outside a tatty arrivals terminal in Spain.

I am not a particularly well-travelled man. I have been all over Europe, bits of North Africa, the famous parts of America. You know, I've been around a bit but I'm hardly Alan Whicker. So, my pronouncements on this sort of thing are not necessarily the most authoritative or credible. But, for what it's worth, north Wales is the most beautiful place I have ever been. Previously, I would have said Lake Como in Italy or perhaps Yosemite National Park in California. But if this was a World Cup of Places (and let's just say it is because that sounds like fun) north Wales would smash the pair of them on the basis that it comprises all the things they have and more. There are astounding views at every turn: all the nostalgic talk I'd heard of sand dunes and forests and golden beaches and awe-inspiring mountains – it was all true. If anything, it was better than even the dewy-eyed reminiscences of my family had suggested.

Even the kids were spellbound. We all were. There was something about it that lifted our hearts. We didn't do anything special. We just hung about with massive smiles on our faces for a week then drove home to London feeling happy and rested.

Where we stayed, in a small village just north of Barmouth, there was Wi-Fi and flat whites and all the other bollocks that used to be the preserve of urban life. As a vegetarian, I was slightly concerned that I might be ill-catered for while eating out. But even that turned out to be city-folk prejudice: at a deli next to Harlech Castle, I bought a vegetarian Scotch egg encased in onion bhaji rather than meat. That's right! A hard-boiled egg inside an onion bhaji! It was one of the most delicious, not to mention innovative, snacks I have ever tasted.

I don't suppose they would have had those sort of mod-cons back in the seventies. But still, how could my parents have divorced after visiting a place as wonderful as north Wales?

Being in nature has become hugely important to me. It's analogous to the awakening I have had in middle age. The beauty was around me all the time – I just hadn't been paying attention. But now I do. Every day I spent time among trees and birdsong and it was a guaranteed mood-cleanser.

A few times a year, I go away with my cousin Bruce on a walking weekend. We pick an area where there are plenty of shaded woods, coastal paths and undulating hills and just get at it for a couple of days. Both of us live and work in cities and we find it helps to get out of the buzz, noise and pollution once in a while. We are dads with bills to worry about, kids to feed and deadlines to hit. Like everyone else, life gets on top of us. Sometimes we must run away from it for forty-eight hours. But boutique hotels or luxury spas just seem like throwing good money after bad. A cheap Airbnb in the middle of nowhere offers better value. Nature is good for you, it's free and it is everywhere.

The practice of *shinrin-yoku* or 'forest bathing' has been prescribed by doctors in Japan since the eighties.

Back then, people were becoming more aware of the depression, distraction, aches, pains and general malaise caused by urban living. Going for a slow walk in the woods combines the benefits of meditation, mindfulness and exercise in a less intimidating form. Mindfulness is difficult. Exercise is exhausting. Meditation is boring. But anyone can go for a stroll through some trees. Just by absorbing the gentle sounds, fragrant smells and beautiful sights of the woodland, strung-out city dwellers can experience immediate mental and physical benefits. To do it properly, you're supposed to leave all electronic devices at home, proceed at a calm pace and embrace the silence. But Bruce and I have got our own twist on *shinrin-yoku* which involves talking bollocks along the way.

From the high-minded (politics, literature, art and the sciences) to the trivial (football, biscuits, cats, fights in pub car parks) we exchange ill-informed, confused and pointless opinions on pretty much anything. We do it partly to amuse ourselves and each other. We've been doing it since we were kids. We used to do it in the garden at our grandma's house; then we graduated to doing it over beers in the pub. Now we find we are able to talk just as much brilliantly mindless shit as ever, even though we are now a couple of sober, middle-aged farts. It's about more than just making each other laugh. It is genuinely cathartic to check out of the mundane practicalities of everyday adult life and let your mind run free for a bit, just like it did when you were a kid and still had a real imagination.

Grown-up life – with all its dreary obligations and responsibilities, its humdrum to-do lists, its soul-crushing repetitiveness and its saddening predictability – can be really tedious. It is cleansing and therapeutic to activate your brain's scattergun mode, allowing your thoughts to roam to strange and unusual places and conjure ideas that aren't practical or necessary but just daft and joyous. Being with a mate who likes doing the same sort of thing is brilliant: you almost compete to see who can talk the most shit and remind each other that you were once both children who didn't feel obliged to have lucid opinions on the situation in Ukraine or strategies to reduce your mortgage repayments.

Doing this while puffing your way up and down hills, past trickling streams and through enchanting beams of sunlight that dance through the leaves and bracken, is a profoundly powerful form of self-care. The stillness of the environment is comforting. It massages the mind and the senses tenderly, helping to bring out the stupid crap that has been lying around at the back of your brain for ages, like a forgotten-about jar of pickles on the top shelf of the fridge. Plus, there is no one else around to hear the bollocks you're chatting when you're deep in the woods. We walked fifteen miles through the Hastings Country Park on a Saturday in early summer and only encountered about three other people along the way. We nodded kindly at them, in the way hikers do, pressing pause on our moronic conversation until they were safely out of earshot. The squirrels and butterflies we saw didn't judge us for the rubbish coming out of our mouths. At least I don't think they did. We were just two men in our late forties, imbibing the breathtaking majesty of Mother Nature while arguing about the merits of the new white-chocolate digestives by McVitie's.

It was life affirming, soul cleansing and beautiful. If you want to get your head straight, hit the woods with a mate who likes to talk a right load of bollocks. *Namaste.*

On New Year's Eve 2023 I stayed in, watched telly and fell asleep at 10 p.m. It was lovely. When I woke up the next morning I felt at peace because I knew that I was living free of the New Year Curses: hangovers and resolutions.

Making resolutions is like making long to-do lists: you're setting yourself up to fail. Planning for a bulletproof, high-achieving, relentlessly happy twelve months is insanity. My only ambition at the start of a new year is to just keep going. There will be bad days, there will be good days, there will be moments when everything looks hopeless and other times when life just seems to breeze along nicely with you barely noticing – like one of those sweetly struck volleys that you hardly feel leave your boot before it ripples the net (I've never actually hit one of those personally but I've heard people talking about them).

No matter how much you plan, life will always meander unpredictably and kick you in the bollocks when you're least expecting it. Your only resolution can be to roll with the punches as best you can, savour the good moments (without letting them go to your head) and have faith that the bad moments will eventually pass.

I find it helpful to look out for the tiny pleasures in the everyday. If you get a buzz off a nice cup of tea, a jog round the park, a once round the living room with the vacuum while listening to the Pointer Sisters on your headphones, then you'll never be short of the odd smile. Sorry if that sounds like twee bollocks but it honestly is the sort of stuff that steers me through difficult times.

Chapter 10

Stop Shitting Yourself
About Talking

Most people who knew me in the past (before I went barmy and started spouting all of this mental health stuff non-stop) would have thought I was a right carefree Jack the lad without a trouble in the world. Clearly, that was an act designed to protect myself.

When I started writing about these sorts of issues, I drew upon a lot of detailed experience from my personal life. I felt as if I could only explain the way I felt by describing the experiences I'd had. Including some painful memories that involve people I love. It's not always big, dramatic incidents. Very often it's seemingly little things that people said or did to me when I was younger – an insult, a joke, a throwaway remark – that secretly scarred me for ever. I'm hoping to help other people see that these small things that might have hurt you when you were young are nothing to be ashamed of. Instead of trying to repress them, you should acknowledge them, try to understand them and, eventually, move on.

It's tough writing about people I love in a truthful way without potentially causing offence or hurt. What I've tried to do is look at every incident, argument, conflict or moment of trauma from the other person's perspective as well as my own. Almost always, I can look back and see that the other person was hurting in their own ways and, like me, had developed elaborate ways of hiding their pain.

Sometimes, carrying secret pain inside can make you act like a bitter, angry arsehole. It happens to the best of us. I've had really close people do the right dirty on me in the past. Writing about it has helped me understand why they did it. It's helped me to forgive and move on.

Another challenge is writing stuff that I know my kids will probably read one day. Like stuff about my drug taking. So I've taken both of them aside, on separate occasions, to give them a heads up. They've been very interested in and highly supportive of my writing. It was easy for me to tell them about some of the content.

My daughter is a teenager and therefore hardly a stranger to drug chat. She was very relaxed when I told her about the fact I used to take drugs. In fact, she didn't seem in the least bit surprised, to be honest. She knows it's all in the past and, I think, is pleased to have a dad who is now teetotal. If only because I can provide late-night lifts on Fridays and Saturdays for all her friends.

As for my son, who is a bit younger, he seemed bored by the discussion. He likes talking about football, space and travel. Chatting about my shameful past of boozing and drugs just feels like wasted time to him. In any case, I've told him to come back to me with further questions whenever. As yet, he shows no desire whatsoever.

I like my kids to know I'm a bit flawed and vulnerable. So many of us put our parents on a pedestal (I know I always did) and when we find out about their imperfections later in life, it comes as a terrible shock. My kids know I'm human and it doesn't seem to bother them. It just gives them more material to take the piss out of. Good luck to them.

Most men don't realise they're suffering from a mental health issue until it's almost too late. They deny themselves self-reflection and just don't think they deserve to feel shit. But we all feel shit. The trick is to own up about it, first to yourself and then to others. So my message to everyone is: take a breath, recognise your feelings and go easy on yourself.

I was doing a radio show around 2008. A comedian I vaguely recognised was one of the fellow guests. He was funny and likeable. Amid our off-air chat, he kept making light reference to the fact that he hadn't worked in a while due to his mental health. I felt really awkward and sort of pretended not to have heard those parts of the conversation. I wanted to keep talking about football and comedy and other pointless shit. I didn't want to hear about his problems; they made me feel uncomfortable and I didn't know what to say.

When we got on air, I became very nervous about him bringing up the subject of his depression because I thought it would make for awful radio. I figured people switched on the radio for a bit of light entertainment, not dark and twisty ruminations on a sad comic's inner life.

What different times they were. This was all a good few years before I hit my own bumps in the road (by which I mean suffered depression, became immobilised by anxiety, turned to drink and wound up with a bastard coke habit before seeking therapy and sorting myself out). It's a shame that I had to go through those shitty experiences to recognise the importance of talking about my mental health. It's a catch-22 situation: you don't like talking about your feelings, so they ferment, mutate and send you mental. Eventually (with any luck) you realise help is out there and you start to share. And then you realise that sharing was what you should have been doing all along. Because getting stuff off your chest is cathartic and discovering that you have the love, understanding and kindness of people around you is life changing.

The biggest barrier for most blokes, I reckon, is shame. We look around and hear stories about people with trauma and depression and often think, *What the fuck have I got to be sad about?* But to imagine that mental health problems are reserved for a small number of deeply troubled individuals is wrong.

It's not about who deserves to feel sad. It's about being human. None of us are immune to feeling shit from time to time. The important thing is to recognise it before it gets out of hand. If you're busy and all of life's little stresses and strains are mounting up, allow yourself to acknowledge it. Take a step back and talk to someone. It doesn't have to be an earnest chat; it needn't be weird and you shouldn't worry about seeming needy. 'I'm having a shit week,' really is enough. Tell your mates, your partner, your family. Get used to chucking it into conversations. You will probably be surprised by the understanding you receive.

Most importantly of all, recognise these feelings in yourself. Stop beating yourself up for feeling shit. It's the most normal thing in the world and there is help out there.

Chapter 11

Stop Shitting Yourself
About Booze

I started writing and talking about being sober publicly a few years back because I wanted people who are in the same situation that I was once in to see that there is a way out.

I was a fucking mess in my late thirties. Too many years of pouring myself into the pursuit of ambition, achievement, excitement and distraction had taken its toll; I had never stopped to process the things that had shaped me, the feelings I thought, who I was and who I really wanted to be. My life was being guided by a warped and synthetic idea of masculinity and success. It was confusing, tiring and depressing, and I started using booze and drugs to cope.

Every day something reminds me of what a good decision I made back in 2015, when things had got a bit too chaotic and miserable for me to cope with. I needed to improve so many different aspects of my life: my relationship with my wife, my performance as a dad, my physical fitness, my mental health, my career, my financial situation and my increasingly volatile emotions.

It felt like such a lot: like a drawer filled with a tangle of charging cables that look like they could never be undone. But it turned out the solution was simple: all I had to do was stop drinking. I was smart enough, strong enough and surrounded by enough love and support to get everything sorted. I just needed to get sober first. Nine years on, I am so grateful that I took the plunge and decided to quit for good. To get back on track I needed to remove the option of booze for ever. I want others to see that there is a way out. I don't think I am any smarter or stronger than the next person. I just woke up to the fact that booze was the common factor in my problems. I am proud of what I did. I don't want to ever get complacent about it or lose sight of the fact that it plays a massive role in everything that's good about my life.

I still have shitty days just like anyone else. But I feel so much more able to cope with them now. I know myself better, I'm braver about facing down challenges and more acutely aware of the good things that surround me every day. Those things – chief among them my relationship with my wife and kids – offset the bad. I feel like sobriety flushed the fear and cynicism out of me, enabling me to enjoy life more and more with each passing year.

It was summer 2023 and I had just turned eight years sober. I was watching the Arctic Monkeys on TV at Glastonbury with my family on a warm Saturday night with the back door open and the cool breeze wafting over us gently. Just my wife, my daughter, my son and me, all slumped together on the sofas, eating, laughing, taking the piss out of each other. I try not to overthink those moments but I did take a breath and reflect a little bit on how safe and relaxed and surrounded by love I felt. I didn't feel proud. I felt lucky and grateful.

I was delighted that my kids derive as much pleasure from music as I do. I felt so lucky to have shared that love with my wife all the years we have been together. But most of all I just felt proud and happy that I could sit and enjoy the performance without picking holes in it, moaning, or writing snide stuff on Twitter to get attention. I just sat back and absorbed it with a smile on my face, then went to bed. That, in a nutshell, is what sobriety has done for me. If you're curious, give it a go. You might like it.

I know that when I was still boozing, I would sometimes see sober people going on about this sort of stuff and think, Fuck off you boring, smug twat. And I'm sure that's how I might come across to some people. But it doesn't matter because this isn't aimed at those people who love drinking and have no desire to stop. I wish them well – I'm not by any means against having alcohol if it makes you happy. These messages are only aimed at those who feel like I did in my late thirties: scared, lonely, desperate to stop but unsure of how to go about it.

The first step is working out if you actually have 'a problem' or not. Doctors, therapists or internet questionnaires might try to establish this by asking questions such as: 'Do you struggle to just have a couple? Do you think it's a bit boring to stop at one? Do you ever drink just to alleviate boredom? Is alcohol inextricably linked to relaxation, fun, excitement, celebration and commiseration? Or do you just like the taste of it?'

But none of it really matters. The only thing that matters is how you feel about your drinking. Do you want to keep doing it? Then keep on doing it, I guess. Unless people close to you are begging you to stop. But, even then, you have to ask yourself if you only want to stop just to appease them. Do you value booze more than your relationship with other people? Are you OK with maybe losing people as long as you can keep drinking? Then keep going.

If you'd really like to stop but are finding it difficult to do so, then I would call that a problem. Personally, I spent a couple of years repeatedly resolving to quit drinking, then falling off the wagon and feeling shit about myself.

When someone eventually told me that my only option was to stop completely and for ever, I was really open to that idea. I had tried cutting down a million times and it never worked. Once you've crossed that invisible line into problematic drinking, just a taste of booze will trigger a thirst that feels insatiable. In my late thirties my resistance to the effects of drink increased rapidly. As a result, my consumption started to spiral. With me, it was a case of all or nothing. So, in the end, I chose nothing. It wasn't easy – especially to begin with – but eventually I came to see that being sober wasn't about the stuff you sacrifice but the stuff you gain: like energy, focus, better health and fitness, increased creativity and mental spark, improved engagement with your loved ones, a turbo-powered ability to feel fulfillment in everyday life and – best of all – love.

Drinking, ultimately, made me sloppy, cynical and dull. It made me harder to love. It made it harder for me to show love to others. Sobriety allows you to open your heart and rediscover how much fun life is. Look at kids: those little bastards are almost always laughing and loving life. And they're never pissed. At least I assume not.

Some drinkers hit rock bottom: a desperate state where they have fucked things up so badly that their need to get help is self-evident. But I think it's just as hard (if not harder) to be stuck in a grey area: not quite getting nicked for public indecency, pissing your pants at work or losing your family, but nonetheless unable to function happily without drink inside you. It's confusing if you have a family and a career and all the other facets of supposedly civilised life but also drink every day to cheer yourself up. You might feel like your relationship with booze feels a bit iffy but society is not quite judging you for it yet, so you have no incentive to stop.

This was where I was at once. I never committed to AA full time or went to residential rehab. I got some therapy, changed my habits (initially in small ways) and tried to constantly look for the positives in sobriety. It worked.

When I was a teenager I think I aspired to have a drink problem. We all drank. But in my youthful search for identity, I decided that it would be cool if 'liking a drink' defined me somewhat. I figured I needed a big statement to establish my credentials as a Keith Richards figure amongst my peers. But I realised that claiming to have sclerosis of the liver or 'wet brain' might seem a bit implausible for a sixteen-year-old. Then, one day, I developed a mild condition whereby it felt uncomfortable to swallow food or water. It was a bit like a sore throat. I went to the family GP (an eccentric quack who once prescribed my brother 'brandy and sausages' to help him gain weight and become more 'robust') and he said there was nothing wrong with my throat. He speculated that it might be a condition called 'raw gullet' which was usually the result of an unhealthy lifestyle.

'Could it be related to alcohol?' I said, excitedly.

'Possibly.' He shrugged.

And that was it. I left the clinic with a spring in my step, eager to tell all my mates that a medical professional had diagnosed me as a problem drinker who had eradicated the lining of his gullet (whatever the fuck that is) through excessive, wildman boozing. None of my mates was impressed, of course. They pissed themselves laughing and immediately started referring to my illness as irritable bowel syndrome (particularly in front of girls). My bid to rebrand myself as a dangerous addict on a runaway train to oblivion completely backfired.

I deserved the ridicule, of course. What sort of prick tries to spread a rumour about himself being an alcoholic? The sort of prick who has been raised in an environment in which alcohol consumption is synonymous not with misery but with glamour. The sort of prick who had been searching for an alluring identity throughout his adolescence and had been bombarded with messages from family, friends, TV, pop music and movies that suggested 'hard drinker' was the best one out there. What's more embarrassing is the fact that I didn't manage to let go of this childish aspiration for another twenty-four years after the 'raw gullet' episode. I never managed to step back and look at life in a broader sense, understand that there were infinite lifestyle choices, sources of pleasure and avenues to happiness and wellbeing that didn't involve chucking alcohol down my throat every single night of the week.

The culture that surrounds us is pretty mental. When I was a kid, the biggest icon for lads like me was Paul Gascoigne: a man who was publicly throwing his talent away in favour of life as an alcoholic. When he made a dick out of himself or sabotaged his life yet again, we didn't pity him, we didn't empathise, we celebrated him. 'Go on, Gazza, you fucking legend!' He was not living life on his own terms. He was enslaved by booze. He was living life by the terms of a culture that says you can't have fun or relax without drink. A culture that says hard drinking is masculine, cool and exciting.

Not much has changed. When Man City won the Champions League in 2023, the media and football fans alike clapped like seals at the sight of Jack Grealish pouring neat vodka down his throat in celebration. The other players, sober and measured in their responses, were labelled 'robots'. Grealish, pissed off his nut and acting the goat, was referred to as 'more human'. Fucking hell.

To get sober and stay sober, you need to start questioning all this bollocks. You need to break free of the glib cultural messaging that hoodwinks you into choosing booze as a central part of your identity. You need to have the courage to show the world that you can still be one of the lads without being twatted. Or just don't be one of the lads if you don't want to be. After all, it can get boring sometimes.

One of my biggest fears when I quit drinking was how I would explain myself to people.

'I'm just taking a break.'

'I try not to drink between Sunday and Thursday.'

'I'm on antibiotics.'

These are the sort of limp, bullshit excuses I used to wheel out when people asked why I wasn't drinking. It made it really easy for them to say, 'Don't be boring, just have a pint.' And it was all too easy for me to cave in. I wasn't being honest about my drink problem. I was playing it all down to make myself feel less ashamed, make others feel less awkward and protect myself from people taking the piss. I was worried that claiming I had a serious problem would come across as a little bit 'extra'. That people might think I was being over-dramatic or seeking attention. I also feared that announcing that I was attempting to get sober for good would mark me out as a boring weirdo.

I wish I'd known then what I know now. Firstly, that no one really gives much of a shit about anyone else's drinking habits. Some mates might take the piss a bit the first time you talk about it in the pub but ultimately it's quite boring and everyone's got their own shit going on. Secondly, the only person who can judge your relationship with booze is you. It's not for others to tell you if you have a problem or not. How could they know? I opened up to a couple of mates when I suspected I was an alcoholic and they laughed, told me to chill out and ordered me another pint. The last thing they wanted to believe was that I was an addict. Because if I was, maybe they were too . . . Once I had established in my head that my drinking was out of control and that I wanted to find a way of quitting for ever, I had to make myself accountable. Embracing accountability is the most important and powerful step you can take when you first quit drinking. Without it, you will really struggle to sustain your sobriety long term.

But what does accountability really mean in this context and how do you enact it? My addiction therapist explained it to me like this: you have to remove your 'secret doorways'. That means denying yourself the little get-outs that have always allowed you to fall off the wagon without it feeling like a big deal. If you tell everyone you're just taking a short break from booze or some other poxy excuse, you are playing it down. This means that it's easy to just say 'Ah, fuck it' and have a drink the moment the urge starts to get the better of you.

If you make out to everyone that you don't really have an issue with booze, you're in control and you're not seeking to quit, then nobody will really notice or care when you fall off the wagon. You won't have to feel any embarrassment or sense of failure when you reach for the bottle. People are likely to cheer you on when you do so. These are secret doorways you leave ajar for yourself whenever you resolve to quit drinking. They are the comforting plan Bs that mean it doesn't really have to be for ever.

They condemn you to failure. As long as they exist, I believe the lure of drink will always get the better of you. You will always be able to tell yourself that having a couple of cheeky pints won't harm you or anyone else. But, in my own experience, getting stuck in that endless cycle of abstinence, relapse and guilt is extremely painful, boring and frustrating. It can scratch away at your soul.

You have to make yourself accountable. That means eradicating all those secret doorways. It means making a real and explicit commitment to yourself that you want to stop drinking. That you know your entire life will benefit from it. And that you're backing yourself to make the change. Don't sugarcoat it. Don't tell yourself that it's only because you want to sleep better or lose a few pounds. Accept that drinking is making your life shittier and sobriety will make it much, much better.

Slam the next secret doorway shut by telling everyone about your decision. Do it with pride, honesty and clarity. It doesn't have to be dramatic or self-indulgent. Just blunt and direct.

'Why aren't you drinking, mate?'

'Because I've quit alcohol.'

'What? Completely? Why?'

'Because I had a drink problem, it was making me miserable and so I decided to stop for ever. Mine's a Heineken Zero, please.'

You'll be surprised how respectful people are when you are as clear and direct as that. If you tiptoe around the subject, play down your decision or take the piss out of yourself for being 'boring', other people will take your lead and take the piss back. But if you are proud and transparent people will take you seriously, respect your decision and stop bothering you about it. At least most will. Those that do give you grief probably aren't worth your time or energy. Quitting drink can be a great friend filter in that way.

I feel like I should repeat the fact that all this advice is only for people who really feel like booze is making them unhappy or costing you more than money. I understand that the majority of drinkers enjoy it as a simple and harmless pleasure. But if you do feel you have addictive tendencies and that one never seems to be enough, then I can highly recommend complete abstinence. By harnessing the all-or-nothing mentality that made you drink too much, you can actually become addicted to sobriety quite quickly. Don't wait around to get started: fuck your mate's stag. Fuck your brother's birthday. Fuck that holiday in Spain. Do them sober. You'll still have fun at all those things sipping on a zero per cent beer because you are a fucking legend. You just won't have a hangover the next day.

Here is an example of what life is like in sobriety. I don't go out nearly as much as I used to but, when I do, it's got to be for something genuinely appealing (not just random Wednesday-night drinks). It was an August evening and I was going to meet my wife. I like to approach these things properly so I ironed a top, had a shave, walked to the tube station, went up west and the two of us went for a bit of dinner. I was not late. I was not talking too loudly, slurring or repeating myself. I was the good company my wife deserved. Then she took me to a fancy work party at a swishy bar full of her colleagues.

Everyone was bang on the booze at this do. Someone asked why I was sipping a glass of fizzy water. The obvious answer was, of course, 'Because still water is for squares.' But I didn't say that. I said what I always say, 'Because I was a massive pisshead so I had to stop drinking booze for ever.' Sometimes that amuses people. Sometimes it freaks them out. Either way, it does a good job of preventing any further questions.

Publishing is a bit of a boozy industry. But then again, what industry isn't? I'm always amazed by the amount of people who claim that their industry is the reason for their unhealthy relationship with alcohol. 'Oh, well, I'd like to cut down, but you see it's so difficult in my industry because everything centres around booze . . .'

Yeah? Join the club. Your industry isn't anything special, wild or glamorous. It's just work. Most work sucks and booze is a popular way of relieving the sense of boredom, exhaustion and despair it generates within your soul. Doesn't matter if you're an accountant, the lead guitarist in Mötley Crüe or a carpet fitter, you will constantly find yourself in situations where booze is made available to oil the wheels of the grind.

People often assume that it was my life in the media that drove me into addiction. It wasn't. In fact, work responsibilities usually made me temper my bad behaviour (with only the odd, notable exception. Like when I got hammered at a banquet for a visiting delegation from the Chinese government and sang, 'I'm forever blowing bubbles' in front of them. To be fair, they absolutely loved it).

Things got out of hand for me when I was bored, lonely and exhausted and started getting solo-twatted in the daytime in a futile bid to make myself feel better. I've never blamed my industry; I've always blamed myself.

Time was, I would have been firing into the free alcohol on offer at a party. Standing about making conversation with strangers can seem awkward and difficult; a couple of stiff ones can lend a helping hand. It all seems quite innocent until you're banging out a terrace anthem in front of 150 bewildered communist bureaucrats.

All I can tell you is, I had a great time sober at that do. It's all I'm used to now. Once you've done pissed things sober a few times you realise it's easier, cleaner and more fun that way. You come to understand that you are able to be interesting, energetic and convivial in the company of other people without having to drink a magic potion first. It makes you feel good about yourself.

If you get bored, it's not because you're sober. It's because the situation is boring. So go home and do something less boring instead. Don't rely on booze to make shit things good. Just avoid doing shit things.

I first understood the idea of alcoholism via watching Sue Ellen on *Dallas*. She had a major voddy habit and was forever straining to resist another glass, her hand shaking as she reached out slowly, mascara streaming down her face, JR Ewing cackling at the spectacle of his own wife's hopeless addiction. I assumed that was what it was like to be a recovering addict: forever caught in a torturous purgatory where the one thing you desired was the same thing that would kill you. Turns out, recovery can be a whole lot more pleasant than US soap operas from the eighties would have us believe.

The last drink I had was in June 2015. Prior to that day, there had been relapses. Dozens of them, maybe more. I had tried and failed to get my bad habits under control for years. It started with me trying to stick to certain boundaries, like never drinking in the week or before 6 p.m. I would succeed in these practices for weeks, sometimes months, but eventually I would go back to drinking arbitrarily.

I even managed to have prolonged periods of sobriety that I thought might last for ever. In 2009 I got a big new job as editor of a magazine and decided that booze and drugs would probably prevent me from doing it properly. I quit completely for about eight months and found it quite enjoyable. The problem was, I never committed to it being a permanent state. I allowed myself the option of falling off the wagon at some point. The fact that I had managed to stay sober for so long gave me the illusion of control. How could I possibly have a problem with drink and drugs if I could so easily do without them for such a long time? I rewarded myself for this achievement by eventually re-embracing intoxication more enthusiastically than ever before. At that stage, I hadn't accepted that alcohol was a problem in my life. I just told people I had taken a break and it was no big deal. That gave me the opportunity to relapse with impunity.

Abstinence is about willpower and, like a crash diet, it's not sustainable. It's about denying yourself something you crave. Often, you end up feeling like you are denying yourself freedom and pleasure. So, inevitably, you relapse. Sobriety is not about willpower. It's more about patience and acceptance. Acceptance that you have no control over your addiction and that it makes your life shit. And the patience you need to learn that life really is so much better without it.

As long as you frame your decision as something you have had to do reluctantly then you will ultimately fail. Accept that booze makes your life shittier and you've got a chance of succeeding. I think people relapse only when they haven't yet accepted the sober version of themselves.

Towards the end of my drug use, I would sometimes try to stay clean for a couple of weeks then cave in after a stressful day and call a dealer. They would deliver the drugs, I would take some and then immediately regret it. In a state of self-loathing, I would throw the rest in the bin. Then, within an hour, I would regret my decision to chuck it away and call the dealer again to deliver some more. I was throwing away more than I took. The dealer absolutely loved it. Mental. And so the cycle of resistance, craving, capitulation and regret would go on and on. Yes, there were clues everywhere that I was not enjoying my habit and that I was not remotely in control.

Ah, well. All's well that ends well, I guess. All I'm saying is, if you relapse, don't beat yourself up too much about it. There is no sober person who didn't fall off the wagon several times before it finally stuck. Treat yourself with a bit of compassion. Know that what you are going through is really hard. But be under no illusion: you are not in control and booze is making your life worse, not better. You're on a lift that is going down. You can't stop it and you can't reverse its direction either. But you can choose to get off whenever you want. Try again. Try harder. Eventually, things will work out.

When I was nine I remember seeing my mum's boyfriend, Rab, bent over the toilet bowl dribbling and moaning. He'd been out at the pub all night, stumbled in after closing and headed straight up to the khazi as usual. I could always hear strange, painful sounding noises when he was in there. But on this one occasion he'd left the door open so I could look upon the troubling spectacle of this bloke – a man who lived with us, who I felt some affection and respect for – heaving and spluttering into the toilet bowl like an animal. It wasn't the indignity of it that really occurred to me at the time. I was just really scared. I ran downstairs and told my mum what was happening. 'Don't worry,' she said, 'he's just had too much to drink.'

My mum wasn't much of a drinker and I don't think I'd ever seen my dad drunk. Rab was a charismatic milkman from Edinburgh who had established himself as my mother's live-in lover and become an entertaining housemate to me but something of a bête noire to my older brothers, who were able to see through his superficial charms and identify him as a bullshitting degenerate. He was the first adult in my life to provide an image of what problem boozing looked like. You might have thought that Rab's alcoholic travails would have put me off for life. But, on the contrary, it was figures like Rab – and numerous hard-drinking peers I met throughout my life – who made it easy for me to slip unwittingly into my own drink problems. As long as I knew drinkers who seemed to be worse than me, I could tell myself I was OK.

I never really felt as if I was one of the worst drinkers in any sphere of my life: in my family, among my pals from school or the people I met through work. I was never even in the Champions League of boozers. I'd have perhaps scraped into the Europa League spots some years. When I was a teenager I made friends with a local pisshead who used to buy me and my mates beers in the local and regale us with miserable tales of how he woke himself up every morning with a can of super-strength cider he kept at his bedside. We didn't regard that as depressing back then; we thought he was a legend. There was another, older pal who used to kickstart his days with a line of charlie off the kitchen counter while his wife was busy getting the kids off to school. One day, his missus caught him and he was so struck by panic that he just ran out of the house without offering an explanation.

I always had mates, relatives or colleagues who would fight, injure themselves or disappear, or just wreak havoc every time they went out on the piss. Me – I'd just be on the sidelines laughing most of the time. I was a funny drunk for the most part, with a tendency to fall asleep before things got too out of hand.

The point is, I never saw myself as having a drink problem because I was surrounded by people who seemed so much worse than me. I chose to use these people as the benchmark for alcoholism. I comforted myself by retelling stories like those above, milking their antics for laughs while creating a flattering contrast with my own modest habits. But, looking back, my relationship with booze was always toxic. I almost always drank to get drunk; I thought nothing of vomiting at the end of the night; I revelled in the sense of anarchy that drink instilled. I got pissed a few times every single week of my life for almost thirty years. It was pretty much my only hobby, my only way of socialising and the only means I had of having fun. By the end, I was unable to have more than a pint or two without the accompaniment of cocaine, and lots of it. Ultimately, I wound up like Rab, a middle-aged man with his head in a stinking toilet bowl while his kids fretted outside the door and wondered what the weird noises were.

Comparing myself to other people completely skewed my perspective on my drinking. It should never have been about how bad I was in comparison to others (especially given that I had grown up around people who were self-evidently functioning addicts). The only thing that should have mattered was how booze made me feel: whether I felt I could control it, whether it was making me happy and how badly it was impacting the lives of those around me. Whether I was drinking a bottle of Scotch a day or just a couple of glasses of wine at weekends, all that mattered was how it made me feel. Whether it was making my life better or worse. Whether it was making me better or worse.

Who gives a fuck how much your mates are drinking? That's their business. The only questions you need to ask yourself are: do I keep resolving not to drink? Do I end up drinking anyway? Does that end up making me feel shit about myself? If the answers to all three of those questions are 'Yes' then you definitely have a problem. If the answer to just one or two are 'Yes' then you probably have one.

I wish I'd asked myself those questions sooner than I did.

Chapter 12

Stop Shitting Yourself
About Other People

When I was a kid Christmas was fucking mayhem. A prevailing state of psychodrama engulfed festivities in the Delaney household. Alcohol and recreational drugs fuelled the dynamic.

A big change happened for me personally around Christmas 1989, when I realised that if I got as pissed as my older brothers, then the situation would cease to seem quite so scary. It was a case of if you can't beat them join them. I joined them when I was about fourteen and didn't look back for the next twenty-six years.

We've got a much younger sister, MJ, who my dad had with his second wife. MJ lived with my dad and her mum in a different part of town. We were all very close, mind you. She would come over to spend a few hours with us in our little council house most years. I remember when my dad dropped her off one Christmas morning, he eyed my brothers and me with grumpy caution. He always regarded us with suspicion and the house we lived in with a thinly veiled distaste. He felt unsure about the wisdom of leaving his pride and joy in the company of his four dipsomaniac sons and his overstretched ex-wife. But leave her he did, knowing that it was what she wanted. And we assured him – PROMISED him – that our much-loved little sis would be perfectly safe in our care.

We were wrong to make that promise. And he was stupid to believe us. Within an hour of him fucking off, my brothers and I were borderline paralytic. By the time my dad came to pick her up in the evening, she was merrily playing with her presents. But my brothers and I were slumped in front of the telly, barely able to communicate properly through the fog of booze and marijuana enveloping our minds. We mumbled and barked at our dad. He expressed disappointment in us, then left.

On Boxing Days, we would all get together at the house of one of our uncles or aunties for a big party with my father's extended family. As I reached adolescence, I would huddle together at these events with the three or four cousins and get surreptitiously drunk on stolen cans of lager. A few years after that we'd be out the back smoking spliffs. A few years later, we'd all be in the bathroom snorting lines. We would celebrate being in each other's company by numbing out the experience with narcotics. I saw my dad's side of the family a couple of times a year for get-togethers in which I often felt uncomfortable. It was a different class environment, a million miles away from the one I lived in day to day. Plus, while there was plenty of love and kindness from all of my relatives, there was also an undertone of bullying dressed up as banter, where the younger kids would be humiliated by one or two uncles and then told to take it all on the chin. There was a big culture of punching down. It was fucking horrible sometimes. No wonder we all started obliterating the experience with drugs and booze as soon as we were old enough.

One year one of my uncles threatened to beat me up in a pub over something I said about Tony Blair. He was drunk out of his mind. As I tried to navigate the situation as best I could (which was not very well at all), other relatives who should have known better cheered him on, willing the physical confrontation to materialise like lunatics at a dog fight. Big crowds of relatives getting together can be lovely but it is also a minefield, especially if booze is involved and a certain number of those present have underlying mental health problems. Unfortunately, this probably describes a great deal of family get-togethers. My advice is to keep it simple: get in, say hello to everyone you need to, load up a plate with as many sandwiches and crisps as you can, then retire to a quiet side room where, with any luck, there might be a TV showing the football.

Having a big family is a real privilege but large gatherings – as pleasant as they are – are rarely the places where real connection with loved ones takes place. Engagement, tenderness, understanding and all the other things that make a loving relationship meaningful tend to unfold in smaller, everyday moments. The mundane minutiae of ordinary life is where love is forged: over cups of tea or swift halves; a catch up on the phone or a warm and unexpected exchange on WhatsApp. It's where we feel better able to show our true selves and what we mean to each other. Christmas or any other big family bash is too big a stage for that kind of thing.

In August 2013 I was flying home from a holiday in Marrakech with my family when my son, who was eighteen months old, began to cry loudly and persistently shortly after take-off, as babies often do. It was stressful and annoying but I had faith that a bit of *Peppa Pig* on the iPad plus a bottle of milk would eventually appease him. There was, after all, a four-hour flight ahead of us.

Then a guy in the seat in front of us turned around and said, 'What exactly is the plan here?' He was a large guy with a beard who looked as if he was in his early sixties. He reminded me of the film director Francis Ford Coppola. At first, I wasn't quite sure what he was talking about.

'What do you mean?' I smiled, while jiggling my son on my lap.

'What I mean is, do you have a plan to stop your kid

from crying or are we just gonna have to put up with this the whole way?' he asked.

Anyone who has ever been a parent of two young kids, sat on a crowded night flight back from north Africa after an expensive holiday that was supposed to relax you but turned out to be just as exhausting as parenting life at home only much, much hotter, will be unsurprised by my reaction.

'What do you want me to do?' I asked.

'Can't you get up and walk him up and down the aisle a bit?' he said.

'Why don't you fucking do it?' I said, holding my infant son out towards him.

'What?!' he replied.

'You heard me, you fucking do it if you know so much about babies.'

'Wait, you want ME to walk your baby up and down the plane?'

'Yes, that's right,' I said. And I tried to hand my son over the back of his seat to him. He recoiled in horror, as if I was trying to hand him a sack full of shit.

He shut up after that, seemingly disturbed by my suggestion. This was a rare case of me responding to dispute or conflict in a way that successfully diffuses rather than escalates the situation. There are only a few moments in life that unfold as if they would in a movie, and this was one of mine.

Mind you, in the spirit of full disclosure, I should reveal the slightly less neat and tidy epilogue to this tale, in which

I childishly pushed and kicked at the back of the man's seat for the rest of the flight. Pathetic.

One of the side effects of neglecting yourself is that you become emotionally volatile. People talk a lot about men getting depressed or anxious but less about the day-to-day temper losses and tantrums that stressed blokes are prone to. These are dangerous and all too common. I've never been a particularly aggressive person – I'm more often than not the bloke trying to stop fights breaking out among rowdier mates. But when I am tired and strung-out I can become grumpy and volatile. Little arguments can blight my day, my week, sometimes even longer. As men, we try to pretend that conflicts and disputes are just water off a duck's back. But all conflict leaves a bruise of some sort. Whether it's a fleeting bit of road rage, a row with an unhelpful call-centre worker or a full-on barney with a judgemental prick on a transcontinental air flight, arguments are horrible. Most of the ones I find myself involved in are avoidable. Taking better care of myself keeps my temper in check and stops me getting so wound up by day-to-day difficulties.

More recently I found myself on another flight with my son, who was by now eleven years old. We were heading for New York in the very cheapest seats available. Leg room was limited and we had over seven hours of confinement ahead of us when the bloke in front of my lad decided to recline the back of his seat to full capacity, knocking a drink off my son's fold-down table and sending his iPad flying. I tapped the man on the shoulder. He turned round, looking as if he had half expected some fallout. I had him down as a serial seat recliner: the sort of bloke who made a policy of trying it on with the passenger to his rear at an early stage of every flight, testing the water to see just how much of the piss he could possibly take.

'Mate, you're crushing my son.'

'Am I?'

'Yes. Plus you just knocked his drink and his iPad over.'

We eyed each other for a moment, contemplating our next moves. It was so early in the flight that any escalation of hostilities could be lethal. I let the silence hang for a while and waited. Eventually he said, 'Well, maybe he could move his seat back as well. Then he'd create extra space.'

I wasn't sure this made any sense, geometrically speaking. More than that, I found it politically offensive. 'But what about the person behind him?'

'Well, they could move their seat back too . . .' he replied.

'Mate, where would we be if we all did the selfish thing and encouraged everyone else to do the same? This is how societies fall apart!'

A look of confusion flashed across his eyes, reminiscent of the bloke on that plane back from Marrakech. Then he said, 'How about we split the difference?' and moved his seat back up by 50 per cent. It was an outcome we were all happy with and reflected on the beauty of pursuing a pragmatic compromise over an unrealistic utopia. In other words, a fine advertisement for the oft-maligned world-view of centrist dads like me.

* * *

I announced on social media that I was publishing a book about mental health, *Sort Your Head Out*, and immediately got a message from an old mate saying, 'Congratulations – but you won't sell any copies.'

Charming!

When you've poured your heart and soul into a deeply personal project for a couple of years, a joke like that can knock you a bit. He wasn't being mean, he was being funny, but sometimes I am a right sensitive bastard.

Oh well, all's well that ends well. The book ended up selling quite a few copies. At one point on its first weekend, it was at the top of the charts on Amazon. There were suddenly a ton of messages in my inbox from people who said that it had encouraged them to open up, show a bit of vulnerability, seek help and perhaps address their drinking. I felt great about that.

When I was struggling in my late thirties, I was ashamed of the way I felt because I didn't think I had the right to be miserable. It would have really helped me back then to know that other people just like me were feeling the same sense of overwhelm. But instead of connecting with people who were going through the same experiences as me, I hid my feelings.

Now if any of this sounds like bragging by the back door, all I can say is that, yes, I am really proud of the writing I have done around mental health. Why wouldn't I be? One of my central messages is that we should all start to treat ourselves with a bit of kindness and try to silence that destructive inner monologue with which we shit-talk ourselves every day.

If you've set out to do something and it's turned out pretty well, then give yourself a pat on the back, for fuck's sake. Self-esteem is hard to come by. Take it whenever and wherever you can. In the past, if I experienced a little bit of professional success, I would have hidden my happiness behind self-depreciation or wild, exaggerated self-congratulation. It was all an act. I just wasn't in touch enough with my own emotions and didn't know how to be sincere.

It works both ways. If you are able to offer praise, encouragement and love while looking someone in the eye, and not dilute it with a silly joke or putdown, you can make a real difference to that person's self-esteem. You also feel better about yourself; it makes you feel open-hearted and authentic. Like you're no longer afraid to show your human side.

Everyone benefits from a bit of love and kindness. Show yourself some once in a while. Whoever you are, I'm sure you deserve it.

I'm a right grumpy bastard sometimes.

I never thought I'd end up like this. Shouting at the telly. Muttering swear words under my breath. Shaking my fist at other drivers. Am I really that bloke now? I asked my therapist about it. 'Why am I so grumpy all the time? Is it an actual condition? Can I get a diagnosis and maybe some pills?' We dug into it and I came to realise that it all stemmed from a mixture of frustration and sensitivity. And that, no, I can't have any pills.

Age has heightened my frustration at the world around me. There was stuff I thought might have changed for the better by now. But some days it only seems to be getting worse. When the Queen died in 2022, I was shocked, then a bit sad but, within twenty-four hours had managed to get grumpy about it. Not at her, but at the reaction of others. The fawning, the performative sentimentality, the perverse nationalism. George Bernard Shaw said that patriotism was the belief that your country was superior to all others on the basis that you happened to have been born there.

I saw another great phrase about this 'national mourning' from a mate on Facebook today: he called it 'the pageantry of subservience'. I grew up hoping that all that bowing down to people who were posher than us would die out in my lifetime. But look at the miles and miles of slack-jawed lickspittles who queued for up to twenty-four hours to pay tribute to the Queen lying in state in Westminster Hall and tell me that civilisation is progressing in the right direction.

See what I mean? I'm a right grumpy bastard. Of course people were upset about the Queen. It was very sad. I probably should have put more time into reflecting on my own sadness instead of condemning others. Shit, I miss her.

In recovery, one of the key things you focus on is letting go of the stuff you can't control. I thought I'd made good progress on that over the years. But there I was getting my knickers in a twist about other people's responses to a stranger's death. What does it matter to me how other people think or feel or behave? It doesn't. Or at least it shouldn't.

Also, I am dead sensitive. I am easily bruised by other people's words and actions. This is ironic because I have always been a loudmouth who perhaps hasn't thought enough about how my words impact on the feelings of others. But there you go. Everyone contradicts their beliefs with their actions once in a while. It's not such a big deal. I'm all for normalising hypocrisy.

Anyway, when a friend, relative or associate says things that annoy or upset me, I can be fucking intolerant about it. Very occasionally, I will confront the culprit there and then – telling them how rude or offensive they've been, explaining the way they have made me feel, perhaps even demanding some sort of apology.

But more often I will put on a phoney show of indifference, then go away and stew on their words for days, weeks, months or years afterwards. My pride stops me from alerting them to the way I feel. I just quietly torture myself about it. Increasingly, I shut myself off from people for long periods of time. I ignore calls and texts. I go out of my way to avoid spending time with them. I let friendships fizzle out without explanation. But because I haven't told them how I feel, they have no idea why I have distanced myself. They probably end up concluding I'm just a grumpy bastard. They'd be right.

All of this bollocks just makes me unhappy. I isolate myself from social situations if I have even the slightest inkling that someone might irritate me. I allow myself to get angry and frustrated about other people's words and behaviours over which I have no control. This is weird, crazy bullshit and I need to get on top of it.

I used to present this current affairs show where a panel of guests would come on every week and discuss the big news stories. The guests were usually comics or journalists and their contributions would be fiery, funny and passionate. But there was one particular guest who became my hero. Whenever I asked her what she thought about that week's topic she would look back at me straight-faced and say, 'I don't care.' This would throw me. What did she mean? She couldn't simply not care. The whole point of this show was for people to at least pretend to care about the subjects we were discussing. I would press her on it.

'You must care!'

'No, I don't,' she would shoot back. Her face was always calm and confident. 'I really don't care.'

We were fucking paying her for this! It was alarming. It was unique. I absolutely loved it. In a world filled with hot air, angry invective and contrived passions, she had weaponised indifference. I asked her back on the show again and again because I found her attitude so captivating. Now I think of it as inspirational too. My life would be so much better if I gave less of a shit about stuff. At least the stuff that doesn't really matter. I just need to work harder at identifying what that stuff is, I guess.

I am not alone in being a grumpy bastard, of course. They are everywhere, and it can be dangerous. We are a moody nation as it is. We're not like those Americans with their bright, white perma-smiles and deranged sense of optimism. Or the Scandies with their irritatingly measured air of intelligent contentment – like a nation of modestly successful architects. Even the French, as grumpy as they seem, have their philosophy to fall back on when life gets rough. When it's cold and rainy outside, they've sworn off the foie gras for Lent and just had to pay a massive tax bill, the Frenchman takes solace in his smug conviction that life is all just an illusion (i.e. the coward's way out).

But we Brits are more straightforward. We say it as we see it. There is no grand notion guiding us through the turbulent patches of our dreary existence. When things look shit, we accept them as shit and respond accordingly: with anger and self-pity.

I got stuck in one of those yellow-box junctions one morning while giving the kids a lift to school. I drove into the box behind a moving car which suddenly slammed its brakes on, blocking my exit. So, not really my fault but when you're out there in the thick of rush hour nobody wants to listen to your excuses. They beep first, ask questions later. In the three seconds I was stationary in the box, I was angrily beeped at from all angles. I felt like Butch Cassidy at the end of the movie, riddled by the bullets of the Bolivian army.

And the faces that stared out of the car windows: con-torted like gargoyles, consumed by hatred and outrage. One purple-faced man scowled at me and jerked his thumb over his shoulder as if to say, 'GET OUT OF THAT YELLOW BOX NOW YOU DISGUSTING PIECE OF SHIT!' I was a victim of mob hatred. All of these angry, hungry, frustrated people in their slow-moving cars needed an outlet. I provided it. Perhaps their shared animosity helped them feel connected to each other in some small way. Maybe it took the edge off the prevailing sense of loneliness that haunts us all. Perhaps, in that sense, my getting stuck in the box junction for three seconds performed a service. It helped unhappy drivers feel part of something. Feel briefly as one with other human beings. Feel seen.

They would have arrived at work with slightly less rage inside. As a result, they would be easier to be around. Their colleagues would have found them strangely less irritable than usual. Everyone's day would have been slightly, imperceptibly less awful. All thanks to me.

But, please, don't call me a hero. I'm just a grumpy bastard with a car and a short attention span.

It was Saturday afternoon and I was sitting at the dining table having lunch with my family. Suddenly, this woman strolled into my front garden and casually took a seat on the bench in front of the window. She looked older than me, probably in her early sixties, quite smartly dressed and respectable looking. There she sat, dead casual, as if she were in her own front room about to watch *Corrie*. She was separated from us only by the width of the double glazing. I couldn't believe it.

I tapped on the window with my knuckle. She turned her head slowly towards me, seemingly irritated that I had interrupted her nice little sit-down. I gawped at her with an expression that said, 'Do you realise we are sitting here having our lunch?' I was hoping that this was all just a simple misunderstanding: that she had mistaken our garden for a municipal area. But no. She looked straight back at me, eyelids heavy with exasperation, as if to say, 'Chill out, mate, I'm only having a quick rest.' I was bewildered. Sure, I have a bench in the front garden which, I suppose, is a bit of an open invite to weary pedestrians. But there is also a fence that divides my front garden from the street which – I'd always assumed – would make it clear that the seating was reserved for residents and legitimate invitees.

Clearly, she saw things differently.

I waved her away with my hand. Still, she didn't budge. Instead, she held up her hand to me, fingers splayed and mouthed, 'Five minutes?'

At this point, we were just tucking into our sandwiches. We also had a pot of tea on the go (I know what you're thinking, and you're right: we are pretty bloody fancy in my house). All of this would take at least five minutes to consume. I just wasn't comfortable spending that amount of time under the gaze of this uninvited spectator. I waved her away again, this time more vigorously and with a furrowed brow that left her in little doubt as to how serious I was.

Reluctantly, she got up and shuffled out of my garden, then disappeared slowly up the street. The kids looked relieved. For a moment I felt good about my militant stance and the outcome it had secured. I was vindicated. I had prevailed. Then I looked at my wife and she chuckled at me, just a little. My feelings of pride crumbled quickly into shame.

Who was that weary traveller? Why did she require rest so urgently? What would it have cost me to let her sit on my bench for five minutes? It's a stupid bench anyway. No one ever sits on it. We got it off my mother-in-law about eight years ago when she was about to take it to the dump. We thought it would look nice. But it's just clutter, really. At least this woman, whoever she was, was getting some use out of it. Who was I to dismiss her so arrogantly, like King Charles grumpily waving away an intrusive courtier? I should have gone outside and spoken to her. I should have asked if she was all right. Maybe I should have even asked her in for a cup of tea? I panicked. I had become confused and felt strangely threatened. I thought she was taking a liberty.

There's a theory that all acts of violence and aggression are rooted in shame. I've read about how they deal with violent offenders in jail. Perpetrators are invariably triggered by words or actions that make them feel embarrassed; as if someone had made them feel 'less than'. This sense of shame makes them feel threatened and angry. Sometimes, this sparks violence. Thankfully, I'm not really wired that way. At least, I'm not a violent person. But I do get angry when I feel someone is taking the piss. Trouble is, I'm not that good at distinguishing between someone who is taking the piss and someone who is just, say, having a quick sit-down in my front garden.

Anyway, it felt like my own little biblical story: *The Tale of the Knackered Pedestrian and the Selfish Land Owner*. I didn't come out of it looking too good. But maybe it taught me something. The bench has to go.

I received an unsolicited package in the mail. It was a padded envelope, pretty crumpled, my name and address scrawled in Sharpie. Maybe I've watched too many police procedurals, but I immediately analysed the handwriting as being that of a psychopath. I tentatively slipped my finger under the gummed lip of the envelope, mindful that it might harbour traces of ricin or anthrax. I never got over that period in the early-to-mid-noughties where everyone was on constant high alert for powdered toxins sent by terrorists in the post. The breathless news coverage of the time even had my poor old mum opening the gas bill wearing Marigolds, for fear that those crafty bastards over at Al Qaeda HQ might be targeting her.

Anyway, this package. Inside was a slim book, of fewer than one hundred pages. There was no accompanying compliments slip, as I might expect from a publisher looking to elicit a review or favourable comment from an august commentator such as myself. Nothing. Not even a handwritten dedication inside. I leafed through the book angrily, searching for clues – yes, I was angry. I don't like getting stuff in the post, especially when I don't know who it's from. The last unexpected treat I ever received by mail was in 1983, for my eighth birthday, when my aunt Celia sent me a small plastic model of the speeder Luke Skywalker rides through the forest in *Return of the Jedi*. It's all been downhill since then. Nothing but unwanted solicitations from credit firms or grumpy demands from HMRC.

I threw the book on the dining table, where my wife was trying to work on her laptop. 'What the fuck is this?' I demanded. 'Some twat has sent me a book with no note. Is it supposed to be some sort of joke? Or a threat?'

'I'm sure there's some sort of explanation,' she said, calmly examining the offending item.

I charged upstairs to take a (anxiety-triggered) leak, shouting back at her, 'I'm going to burn that book'.

By the time I came back downstairs, she had completed her research and discovered that the book was authored by one 'Samuel Delaney'. 'Oh, I see,' I said indignantly. 'Some joker thinks I might find it entertaining that someone else has the same name as me. How hilarious!'

She reminded me that my grandfather's name was Samuel Delaney. And that, if I'd bothered to read the foreword before losing my temper and resolving to set the modest tome aflame, I would have learned that the book was a short story penned by said grandad several decades ago and discovered by one of my aunts after his death. My uncle had decided to get the story printed and bound and sent a copy out to each member of the family.

The story is set in my grandad's hometown of Newry, County Down, in the thirties, when he was a young man.

After he moved to England and had an inordinate number of children, the original Samuel Delaney worked for many years at the Kodak factory. Writing this short story – which he never showed to anyone – must have offered his sharp and creative mind some form of therapeutic outlet amid the exhausting toil and suffocating responsibility of work and family. It's a shame he never had the confidence to bring it to an audience himself. And it's touching that my uncle made such an effort to bring it to the family's attention all those years later. Ultimately, I'm happy I didn't burn it.

But, for fuck's sake, Uncle, how long would it have taken you to stick an explanatory note in the envelope?

Travelling with the family is stressful. The problem is, my wife and I operate at completely different speeds. She likes to pack days in advance, get to the airport with three or four hours to spare and, once through security, proceed straight to the gate and just sit there, solemnly waiting for the plane to arrive.

I am a nightmarishly casual traveller. I throw things in a bag on the morning of departure, rock up to security about an hour before take-off and then take my time perusing the terminal shops. I'll often buy an unnecessary pair of trainers at JD Sports or a pair of headphones I can't afford at Currys. To me, that's all part of the holiday vibe. Holidays are an act of anarchy. From the moment you leave your house and stick your luggage in the back of the Uber, the usual rules do not apply. For the next week or so you are likely to be wearing swimming shorts at breakfast time and eating octopus for lunch. It's mental, so I try to lean into it. I spend, eat, drink and time-keep as if the world is ending and all actions have no consequence. This is why my wife falls out of love with me every time we set foot in an airport.

The kids have taken sides. My daughter is bang up for shopping and timewasting with Dad; my son is a schedule neurotic like his mum. This divide fuels a toxic, interfamily psychodrama every time we fly. It's awful.

We travelled to Budapest to visit my in-laws. Things got really strange before we even reached Heathrow. The cabbie who drove us there was a talker. I had to sit next to him in the front and he WOULD NOT stop telling me about the varied battery lifespans of electric vehicles. It was very early and I wasn't in the mood. In Germany (where people aren't half as uptight and awkward as we are) Uber gives you a conversation opt-out before your car even arrives. They are such civilised people.

As it turned out, the driver's chatter was only half the problem. As we approached Terminal 3, he announced that he was an accomplished flautist. I made the mistake of expressing mild interest in this, at which point he took out his phone, mounted it on the dashboard and – while we were waiting at the lights – looked up a video of himself on YouTube. In it, he sat in his front room playing a not entirely unappealing Indian folk song. I tapped my foot, nodded my head and just hoped no one in the back started awkward-laughing.

Eventually, we arrived at the drop-off point and my wife, consumed with her usual fears about missing the flight, lunged for the door handle. But the doors were locked. He didn't want us to get out of his taxi. We had seen the video of him playing but that wasn't enough. Now he wanted to play for us in the flesh! With a flourish, he produced a hand-carved bamboo flute from the footwell. 'Just one quick tune before you go,' he insisted. He began to perform a melodramatic ballad that felt as if it lasted for days. It was hot in the car. The driver made unblinking eye contact with me while he played. I glanced at my family in the back: my fourteen-year-old daughter staring at her feet, my ten-year-old son consumed by rage, my wife on the verge of an aneurysm.

Just as I was beginning to contemplate a physical intervention (grab the flute, snap it over my knee and run?), the recital reached its conclusion. The driver beamed at me and waited for a response. I applauded. He was talented, that was for sure. But there is a time and a place for that sort of thing. I'm all for holiday chaos but this was a bit much, even for me. He released the doors and we hurried to departures.

Maybe Uber should offer a flute opt-out.

Every day offers a small adventure or curious diversion like this. The writer Nora Ephron once said, 'Interesting stories happen to people who notice them.' I try to keep an eye out every waking moment. Without it, I might be diverted by the red herrings and straw men that dominated my mind for so many years: the ambition, the hunger for excitement and thrills, the determination to live a life less ordinary. It was all so tiring, so pointless and distracting. I never realised that the brilliance and laughter was already there in the everyday.

It would be very easy for me to withdraw completely from the outside world and just become a hermit. To be honest, I'm halfway there already: I work mostly from a shed in my back garden, dressed all day in elasticated leisure wear. I venture out only to walk the dog and occasionally drive my teenage daughter to and from social events. It's a simple, unfussy lifestyle that I find helps nurture a state of mental balance.

However, I acknowledge that it is also a bit weird and boring. It's also a shame, because I feel as if I still have a lot to offer society: I remain a colourful and entertaining person to interact with, given the chance.

When I do occasionally stray outside my domestic bubble, I always try to make the most of the experience. I am someone who will talk to almost anyone: in the supermarket checkout queue, on the train station platform, even at the urinal at the public loos: if you see me, watch out, because I will try to strike up a chinwag, whether you like it or not.

I was forced to travel to an unfamiliar postcode to pick up some documents from a travel agency. It was a boring, administrative obligation that I was pretty fed up about – until I got to the company's offices and spotted an empty birdcage on one of the shelves.

'Do you keep a bird in this office?' I asked the travel agent.

'Yes, my mother lives in the flat upstairs and has a parrot,' she replied. 'Would you like to see it?'

Had I not asked about the cage, I would have never known about the mother, the parrot or the flat upstairs. You see? I like to chat. It always opens up opportunities. In this case, the opportunity was to meet a parrot and its owner. She was a charming elderly woman who told me her life story while I fed her parrot – Sonny – peanuts through the bars of his cage.

'You're a pretty boy,' I said to Sonny.

'I know that!' he squawked back at me.

It was comfortably one of the top five most thrilling experiences of my year so far. What a cheeky parrot Sonny was.

Eventually, I said my goodbyes and went back downstairs. By now, there was another customer in the office filling out the same forms as I had. I was sure I recognised him. I said 'Hello' in a familiar way and asked if he knew that they had a parrot upstairs. As soon as he opened his mouth to tell me that, yes, he knew Sonny because he was a regular customer, I realised who the man was: none other than noted violinist, celebrity Aston Villa fan and former 'enfant terrible' of the classical music scene, Nigel Kennedy! Still reeling from the excitement of meeting Sonny the Parrot, I wasn't sure if my nervous system was able to process a second shock of this magnitude. For a brief moment, I went dizzy and wondered if I was dreaming. Then I composed myself, told Mr Kennedy that I was a big fan and spent an enjoyable fifteen minutes talking to him about Premier League football.

Back home I told the family, in a state of high animation, of the mind-boggling adventure. They listened to the whole story, spellbound, and I sensed that my wife and kids were starting to see me in a new light. Perhaps I wasn't just the weird, reclusive, unshaven and friendless dope they had previously taken me for. Maybe I was, in fact, a cosmopolitan man about town who hungrily gobbled up the endlessly enriching array of experiences that life served up. A man who could turn a dreary trip to a travel agent into a compelling escapade featuring exotic birds and celebrity musicians. A man who drinks thirstily from life's majestic fountain.

As I concluded, my son commented, 'Sounds like bollocks to me.' My daughter nodded in agreement with him. My wife smiled patronisingly and wandered off.

But it *was* true. All of it. And I don't care if they don't believe me (or if you don't either). Because I lived through it. I had that sensational day out and no one can ever take it away from me. Don't believe what they tell you about Londoners being unfriendly: I'm one and I've been talking my way into other people's lives my whole life.

Being grumpy all the time is exhausting. Getting irritated is really boring. Resenting others is an easy habit to fall into. When you notice yourself drifting in that cantankerous direction, try to connect with people in small ways. Find some common ground. Remind yourself that they are human beings like you, with the same fragility, the quirks, the same flaws and the same brilliant, hilarious strangeness. Engage. Smile. Accept. You might stop feeling annoyed and start feeling a bit more curious.

But if they still seem like arseholes, then they probably are. Just shrug it off and never talk to them again.

Chapter 13

Stop Shitting Yourself
About Your Health

I don't usually weigh myself. What's the point? Owning scales would only make me anxious. The size of my body is just another source of worry. I have generally monitored the fluctuation of my body shape via the fit of my clothes. As long as my jeans still just about do up in the morning, I figure there's no need to panic.

But last week I was weighed at the GP's for the first time in several years. Turns out, I weigh in at an impressive sounding 102 kg. Impressive, that is, if I were a heavyweight boxer formed of sinewy muscle. But I am, in fact, a slightly spongy dad in his late forties with a wobbly stomach. I typed my details into an online NHS thing which told me my Body Mass Index (BMI) was 29.1 and that I had to lose a whopping 5 kg. to reduce my risk of diabetes and heart disease. It was disheartening. It was also surprising. I exercise four or five times a week. I go for long runs and also work out with a personal trainer. I don't drink alcohol. I am vegetarian. I have long since made many of the lifestyle changes most doctors would recommend to anyone trying to take control of their weight. And yet here we are.

I am insecure about this stuff. When I was a kid I was pretty podgy for a few years. I'd like to say this was 'puppy fat' but the truth is that I ate loads of chocolate biscuits and rarely got up off the sofa between the ages of ten and fourteen. The teasing and cruelty that went along with my childhood tubbiness cut pretty deep. The exact wording of insults delivered by bullies, friends, relatives and – perhaps worst of all – secret crushes about my plump appearance still rings vividly in my mind all these years later. This was back in the eighties when sensitivities around weight issues and body image were pretty much non-existent. It was perfectly fine to tell someone you wouldn't date them because they were too fat. Even my absent father once told my mum, struggling to raise me and my brothers alone, that I was too fat and she must take measures to address the situation.

It's hard to get over that stuff. Of course, you can have a high BMI and still be healthy and beautiful and confident. Objectively I know that's true because I can see it in other people. But it's a story that I struggle to tell myself internally with any conviction. I have been slim for most of my adult life. In my late thirties I put a bunch of weight on due to drink. When I got sober I started exercising. Since then I've felt as if I'd got the balance right.

I don't look particularly rotund. I am six foot two and the height manages to hide the weight quite well by stretching it all out lengthways. I'm not massively keen on regarding myself naked in a full-length mirror to be honest (who is?) but I manage to look at photos of myself without feeling too disgusted. I feel fit – certainly a great deal fitter than I did ten years ago. Plus, my blood pressure is healthy and my cholesterol levels are low. Maybe the BMI index is just a scam designed to nurture fear and insecurity in the civilian populace so that we feel ever more dependent on a matriarchal state? You know, like the credit rating system, or Isis.

Yes, I have a habit of second helping at dinner time. I go through phases of rampant chocolate consumption. A Friday-night takeaway is comfortably the highlight of my week. So I realise I am not exactly living the Mark Wahlberg lifestyle. But seriously, what more does my body want from me?

Next, I got diagnosed with sleep apnoea. It's a condition that causes you to stop breathing in your sleep. I know what you're thinking: don't you die if you stop breathing? Well, I'm no doctor, but I think you need to stop breathing for a good couple of minutes to be properly dead. Sleep apnoea generally interrupts your breathing for just a moment or so, causing you to wake up, adjust your sleeping position and drift back off again without even noticing. The worst symptom is that you feel really tired in the daytime. Even if you think you've had a good eight hours, you have, in fact, been awake on numerous, imperceptible occasions. An interrupted sleep like that can leave you not only knackered but – according to the NHS website – irritable and unable to concentrate for long periods.

These are symptoms that are more than familiar to me. So, something had to be done. The GP put me in touch with a local 'sleep professor', who established that I was a big night-time snorer. This, he reckoned, was a dead giveaway to apnoea sufferers. Most apnoea is caused by an obstruction in your airways which tends to grow as you reach middle age and your once beautiful head slowly transforms into a twisted, lumpy mutation, both inside and out.

The prof sent me a test in the post: it required me to stick two small tubes up my nostrils and strap a heart monitor around my chest at bedtime. In the morning, I sent it back to him in the box it had arrived in. A few days later, he called to give me the bad news: I was balls deep in sleep apnoea. But the good news was that he had a cure: a swishy-looking breathing device (real name, CPAP – Continuous Positive Airway Pressure – machine) which gently blows air up your nose while you sleep to keep the old lungs and heart functioning properly throughout the night.

If there are two things I love, it's new gadgets and sleeping. The CPAP machine ticks both boxes, so I was delighted when mine arrived later that week, absolutely gratis thanks to our wonderful NHS (and before any uptight fuckwit complains that this is a waste of resources, you should know that (a) Sleep apnoea really can kill people in their sleep if left untreated and (b) I can't generate the tax contributions that help fund the health service if I'm half-asleep and/or grumpy all day long, can I?).

The device is pretty dainty: it sits looking gorgeous on my bedside table. Inside is a SIM card with a sleep programme created by the professor, just for me. Protruding from the front is a long, concertinaed plastic tube, on the end of which is a plastic mask that sits over my nose and mouth. The mask is held firmly to my face by accompanying head straps. Admittedly, it is not the most elegant of looks to rock in the marital boudoir. But my wife has been very supportive. She laughed a little bit after helping me fit the mask for the first time. But, to be honest, she is a beneficiary of the contraption as much as I am: I was often oblivious to my own loud, incessant snoring. My wife – as she told me regularly and in fairly robust terms – was not.

So now, at night-time, after I've read a few pages of a book, I attach this mad paraphernalia, press the 'Go' button and – somehow – submit to the comforting embrace of what Shakespeare once referred to as 'nature's soft nurse'.

I woke up a few times to readjust the mask, as it took me a while to learn how to tighten it properly to make sure the air didn't blow in my eyes. But now I've got the hang of things and manage to sleep peacefully all the way through. I wake up feeling refreshed and full of pep. My wife hasn't heard me snore for ages. My son says I look like a robot elephant. When I showed him a picture of me with the machine, my best mate said, 'People usually wear stuff like that when they're just about to die.' They've both got a point. But I feel more alive than I have done in years. The last time I felt this energised, I was on drugs.

Given these health concerns, I decided to go for a medical at a private clinic. They do it for middle-aged men like me who want to check that our arteries aren't fucked, our heart's not about to pack up and our prostate hasn't ballooned into a tumour. Plus, they offer a ton of useful health guidance to help future-proof the body. Against what? Hard to say. Death, I suppose. The going rate for this sort of MOT is twelve hundred quid and, for that sort of money, yes, I think I would want to walk away with the secret of eternal life. Fortunately, I have managed to wangle this test for free as part of a journalistic assignment.

After numerous tests, the doctor tells me I am not dying. Or at least I don't appear to be about to die any time soon. My results – the tests on my blood, my heart, my prostate, my muscles and everything else – have been ingested by some sort of health algorithm that compares them to every other bloke of my age in the world and assesses my comparative risk status. This is how medicine works. There is no definitive diagnosis: there are only likelihoods and probabilities, based on comparison. Whether I am strong, fit, healthy, surviving, thriving or dying is defined by context. In this sense, my status is dependent on a giant competition.

I'm not competitive so I don't really like this idea. I don't want to define myself in comparison to others. But this is what being a man can feel like sometimes. It's boring and it's tiring. And I want to opt out.

I took a long, slow run by the River Thames listening to music. Not nosebleed techno. Not the *Rocky* soundtrack. Just some low-key, slightly jazzy hip-hop. Plodding music. The run took me fucking ages but I managed to eke out eight kilometres, my best distance so far that week. My Strava app reckoned I burned nine hundred calories, which I felt good about. I did a bit of work and then, mid-morning, I had a cup of tea with a millionaire's shortbread slice, which Google tells me has about four hundred calories. So I'm still up on the deal. I feel invigorated and content, plus I have a nice sugar rush on the go. This just about sums up my approach to 'Low-Performance Fitness'.

Nowhere is high-performance culture more prevalent than in the world of fitness. Many influencers, experts and celebs endorse goal-driven fitness regimes designed to achieve a specific weight loss, muscle gain or performance target. But all that 'lose two stone in a month' stuff discourages balance and, all too commonly, sets people up for disheartening failure.

I've tried it all in the past. As someone with an addictive personality, all or nothing approaches are attractive.

Years of slothfulness, gluttony and weight gain would be followed by a sudden epiphany, leading to sustained periods of abstinence and super-intense exercise regimes. My weight and fitness fluctuated wildly. My body didn't know whether it was coming or going. My mental health was all over the shop. I lost a couple of stone very quickly after quitting drinking. I cut out all sugar, bread, pasta and rice and started running every day at the crack of dawn. The kilos fell off but I kept getting ill through exhaustion. I couldn't sustain it and ended up putting half the weight back on when it all got too much. The problem was, I felt as if I could only attack fitness plans with an extreme, aggressive mindset. But who wants to be extreme and aggressive all the time? It feels shit and leaves you knackered.

I'm a middle-aged dad with a paunch and a thing for Walkers crisps. I'm not getting a Dwayne Johnson body at my age – I probably never could have had that body, however hard I worked. Our genetic make-up dictates our potential and I come from a scrawny heritage of Irish pissheads and English chip-eaters. There's only so far DNA like that can take you. But I enjoy exercising: it makes me feel good about myself; running is like a form of meditation and lifting weights is cathartic. I box regularly too, which is an excellent way of processing anger and aggression without getting arrested. That might sound like a lot of exercise, but I do it at my own pace and in my own good time. I still eat crisps and sugar. I have pasta for dinner pretty regularly and takeaways are a permanent weekend fixture.

I'm told that weight loss is achieved 30 per cent in the gym and 70 per cent in the kitchen. There is no way you can outrun a bad diet. My diet is half-decent, I reckon. I'm vegetarian and I don't eat many processed foods. But I do believe that eating is for pleasure; being a full-time protein-powder nutter just isn't very attractive to me. I like to eat nice things, often in large quantities. I can't run very fast but I can run for quite a long time. I can't touch my toes. I can lift fairly heavy weights (and even working my way up to that point has taken a good few years).

I have stopped giving too much of a shit about the way my body looks. I just like to do things steadily and often. I don't set targets, although I do like to maintain a vague level of fitness. Basically, I like to feel as if I can run for forty-five minutes or lift weights for half an hour without feeling sick or keeling over. If I feel as if my thirty-four-inch jeans are getting too tight I just cut out the chocolate for a few weeks. I am not trying to cheat death or score points. Fitness just makes me feel good. Lethargy leads to boredom and boredom makes me miserable. Getting my heart rate up first thing in the morning gives me a big lift and tends to make me more productive, creative and efficient for the rest of the day.

Low-Performance Fitness works for me. I'm not a particularly competitive person, even with myself. I'm not that interested in beating my personal best at anything. I'm just happy to keep getting out there every day. Maybe my next book will feature pictures of me sitting on the sofa eating biscuits, then puffing my way through the slowest 10k on record or demonstrating my appalling deadlift technique.

I don't have a problem with the muscle Marys who push themselves further than I ever could. I admire them. But I am sceptical about people who say, 'I did it so anyone can!' Because that's bollocks. We all have different lives, different mentalities, different genes and different priorities. Some of us just choose not to give 100 per cent in the gym. As a matter of fact, I choose not to give 100 per cent to anything. I think that's mad. If you pile all of your energy into any one aspect of your life the other bits are going to suffer and you will lose balance. The most I'll give a job is 60 per cent (and even for that you'd have to pay me really well). I'll give my kids maybe 80 per cent. If I gave them the full hundred I'd only end up resenting them and that would be bad for all of us. Same goes for my wife. And fitness? Maybe 60 per cent in a good week. Life's too short and there are too many indulgences to give it any more than that.

Fitness doesn't have to be extreme or goal-driven. It doesn't even need to be that difficult. You don't have to be any good at it. Just do it anyway. Movement is a magic bullet: it improves everything about your mind, body and spirit. And doing something – however small, rubbish or undignified – is always better than doing nothing at all.

I threw up in a public toilet. It was the first time in years. Still, you never lose the knack. The toilets were in an outdoor car park. They were the kind that require you to pay 20p to gain access. I didn't have any change so I just had to wait outside an occupied cubicle until someone vacated, then I nipped in before the door shut.

Once inside, I quickly fell to my knees and spewed angrily into the stainless-steel bowl. I panted and heaved for a few moments. Then I just stared silently into the bowl and waited patiently until ... another surge of pale-brown vomit gushed forth. My throat retched, my stomach strained, my eyes filled with hot tears. I repeated this stop/start routine a further three or four times before I was spent. And yet, in my mind, I remained calm. It all felt strangely familiar.

Back in my drinking days, this was the sort of semi-regular occurrence that I would have barely noticed. At worst, it would have been an irritating interruption to my day. At best, the basis of a wonderful anecdote for the lads. Either way, vomiting at inopportune moments in unpleasant places was something I accepted as an occupational hazard of the casual pisshead. On this occasion, I was neither pissed nor hungover. I was a forty-eight-year-old father, almost nine years sober, on a short family holiday with his wife and children in the Isle of Wight.

I'd woken up with a bastard of a headache which had only worsened as the morning unfolded. On the drive to a nice little village for an Easter pub lunch, the pain became so intense that it rendered me nauseous. After parking, I told my family to go on ahead of me while I visited the loos 'for a wee'. But I knew what was coming. I was being visited once again, after all these years, by the spew monster. I wasn't scared. I almost relished the prospect. I wasn't fond of the excruciating, undignified and deeply saddening hangovers that constantly accompanied my final years of drinking, but I did quite enjoy the miraculous relief that a hungover chunder would often provide. That feeling of cleansing purge was really quite nice sometimes.

I really hated having a headache so bad that it made me throw up. As I knelt on that toilet floor, I reflected on how much trouble my head had caused me over the years. In fact, I had got so cross and felt so sorry for myself that I had briefly wondered if I'd be better off without the massive fucking thing. Fuck my head. All heads are big. I'm sure I read somewhere that they account for half of the average human's entire body weight (NB, this might be bollocks). But mine is especially large. My mum continues to tell me how the size of my preposterous cranium caused her no end of grief during the birthing process. 'The doctors had to yank you out with forceps in the end,' she says accusingly, as if I had any agency over the matter.

When I was an adolescent I started having epileptic seizures. They continued, on and off, until my mid-twenties and were fucking awful experiences. Once, after watching West Ham beat Derby County 5–1 in the late nineties and then smoking a ton of celebratory hashish in the back of my pal Jasmine's car, I collapsed in the street, cracked my nut open on a wall and suffered a series of epileptic fits that landed me in Kingston hospital for the rest of the weekend. I remember waking up the next morning, still splattered with blood, surrounded by old men who told me that I must have had a heart attack because this was the cardiac ward. I was deeply alarmed. Thankfully, it turned out that I'd only been put in with the codgers with the dicky tickers because of bed shortages elsewhere. 'No need to panic,' said the posh consultant, with a chuckle. 'You're not dying, you just had a massive seizure and cracked your skull open. Better lay off the Moroccan Marlboros!' Charming.

It's not just physical aggro my head has caused. There's all those stupid thoughts it's conjured over the years too: the bad decisions, the relentless worry, the confusion, paranoia, shame, toxic rumination, envy, greed and self-loathing it has been responsible for. If it was an employee, I would have fired it. If it were a girlfriend, I would have dumped it. If it were a mate, I would have probably not said anything but secretly resented it for years before eventually allowing the relationship to just fizzle out naturally.

Plus, on top of all that, it looks stupid. A massive great balloon, wobbling atop my body, painted with an absurd rubbery smile, like an advertisement telling anyone who sees me coming that I am a fucking idiot.

The head is the most ridiculous part of the body. We'd all be much better off without one: the plants and trees seem to do OK. A stomach, a heart and an arse are probably enough to keep most of us happy and out of trouble. Why evolution ever thought to give us a head (and its troublemaking sidekick, the mouth) is beyond me. I wrote my university dissertation on *The Origin of Species* and, I can tell you, Charles Darwin offered absolutely no explanation for the head's existence. Read it yourself if you don't believe me (the book I mean, not my dissertation, which was very dull).

Once I'd finished puking on Sunday, I cleaned up and emerged from the toilet with a renewed vim. Briefly, I knew how Jesus must have felt all those Easter Sundays ago as he swaggered out of his cave.

A glass of fizzy pop and half a breadbasket later, I was back on top form, entertaining the kids with tales of my vomiting antics and shooting the wife a wink as if to reassure her that the horrid old pisshead she had once been married to was gone for ever, and in his place was the sort of practical, can-do husband who was able to brush off a car-park puking incident with a laconic (and sexy) elan.

Shit happens to your body throughout your life and it only tends to get worse as you get older. Despite what high performance nutters might try to tell you, you can't cheat death or reverse the ageing process. But you can do small things to make the life you are living right now slightly more comfortable. Keep moving, quit the fags and try to eat less processed meat for starters. More importantly than all of that, accept that perfection is never possible. That way, you'll at least keep your worrying under control and your mind healthy.

Chapter 14

Stop Shitting Yourself About Being a Parent

My daughter wanted to have her mates over to celebrate her birthday. Sure, I said. But there were some conditions (hers, not mine). She wanted her mum, her brother and me to fuck off out of it for the evening so they could have the house to themselves. Also, she wanted me to lay on a Domino's delivery and some prosecco. What if her mates got pissed and their parents blamed me? No problem, she said. They would stay the night so their parents would never actually get to see them inebriated. A watertight plan.

I found myself saying 'Yes' to everything. It took a couple of days for the absolute pisstake nature of her proposal to really sink in to my tired and weary brain. After which I went back to the negotiation table with some conditions of my own. If she wanted me to lay on booze then there was no way I would be vacating the house. I would, however, get her mum and brother to make themselves scarce.

My wife is a light sleeper who gets a bit, erm, volatile when she is woken. Also, she is far less intimidated by teenage girls than I am. When they stay awake noisily talking all night, it's a nailed-on certainty that my wife will storm in and make a massive scene at least twice during the night. I, on the other hand, am shit-scared of both my daughter and her mates – they would have to be literally on fire for me to enter the same room as them and start issuing orders. Plus, these days, I will sleep through anything. My ability to kip any time, any place, anywhere is magical. I just shut my eyes and – BAM! – I'm straight off to the land of nod, with no chance of even a stir for the next nine hours. Lovely stuff.

I laid on three bottles of prosecco to be shared between seven girls. I figured this was enough for them to feel like they were having a mild piss-up without actually getting pissed up. These girls are amateurs; they have no idea what feeling battered is really like, with all the horror and dread and confusion. But they understandably crave some sense of escape from their tedious and repetitive lives, defined as they are by schools and bus rides, anxious parents and strung-out teachers, meaningless rules and existential dread.

One day they will learn that the only way to cope with these daily assaults on their emotional wellbeing is to face them head on, not try to escape into the corrosive oblivion that alcohol provides. But I can't explain all that to them now. It would make no sense. They have to try this shit out and, hopefully, come to understand the futility of it all for themselves. Until then, I'll buy them their cheap bubbly wine and get a couple of jumbo pepperonis delivered to the door for them to soak it all up with.

On the night of the do, I packed my wife and son off to the mother-in-law's, then locked myself in my bedroom with a bag of salted pretzels and a bottle of zero per cent lager. While I watched *Midsommar* – a profoundly disturbing drama about a batshit Swedish cult – I heard occasional shrieks and whoops from downstairs. I didn't go down to investigate. These are good kids. What's the worst that could happen? I'm teetotal and my wife barely drinks. There is no alcohol in the house for them to raid beyond what I bought specifically for the party. I let them get on with it.

When I was their age, I was out and about guzzling booze in parks and on the streets, completely unsupervised. Most parents back then forbade alcohol so everyone had to do it in secret. I'd like to say it didn't do us any harm but, thirty years later, I ended up in addiction therapy, so . . .

What's the solution? Hard to say. Prohibition doesn't work: it just drives teen drinking underground. Allowing them to do whatever they like is a risky strategy too.

Keeping it within the confines of the home – with a semblance of control over exactly how much booze they can access – seems the safest bet.

I can report that none of them puked or died and they'd all gone home by ten the next morning so I'm chalking this one up a victory. I like to think of it as iron-fist-in-a-velvet-glove parenting. One–nil to me.

* * *

It's a wet, warm morning in late August. I'm sitting in my car outside the school, worried about where my daughter is. She walked through the gates almost an hour ago with her mates to collect her GCSE results. My wife and I are waiting outside for back-up purposes: under strict instructions to keep a safe distance but be ready to provide emotional support should things go wrong.

I tap at the steering wheel anxiously and study the faces of other kids emerging with results papers in their hands. Could their expressions offer clues to what's going on inside? Why is my daughter taking so long? Is that a good sign or a bad sign? 'I think it's a good sign,' I tell my wife. 'If it was bad news I think she would have shot straight back out to see us.'

My wife doesn't respond. She is relaxed about the whole thing. She has faith, I guess, that the results will be good. Or that, even if they aren't, everything will turn out OK. Our daughter will cope. It won't be the end of the world. We'll work out what to do next and life will go on. Sometimes, being married to someone so rational and calm can be as annoying as it is reassuring. Mind you, I don't suppose it's as annoying as being married to a neurotic like me, who responds to moments of tension by pathologically filling silence. I begin to describe my own GCSE results day, thirty-two years previously, at the very same school. Only I didn't go to the school to collect the results. I was on holiday in Europe and had to get my mum to read them out to me over a crackly phone line from England. 'I think you got a kkkkkkzzzzzzz crackle-crackle in biology and, um, let's see, a ffffffffzzzzzz crackle fffffzzzzzz in English . . .'

Examination boards sent your scores to your home address on little slips of paper. It was confusing. That, combined with the sketchy state of pre-internet continental phone lines, meant that I wasn't quite sure if I had passed or failed any of my subjects until I got home a couple of weeks later. I hadn't expected to do well. I ended up doing well enough to qualify for my A-levels. Once it was all confirmed I remember a feeling of unprecedented lightness and optimism. I had hardly smashed it but I at least knew I had done enough to open the next chapter of my life. I could stop worrying for a short while. Until the next uncertainty came along. Life has pretty much stayed that way ever since: an endless cycle of worrying about the future punctuated by the occasional respite, in which life seems fleetingly safe and predictable. Now I'm just always happy to know I've got the next mortgage repayment covered, to be honest. I don't have time to think about the bigger picture.

My wife, who rarely got below an 'A' grade in anything, has no detailed recollection of her GCSE results day. Nor her A-level results day, her university graduation or any other moment of achievement in her life. I find this strange: I can usually recall the sounds, the smells, the shoes I was wearing, the prevailing weather conditions and everything else about every significant episode I've ever experienced. Maybe because the fear and tension I feel makes me hyper-vigilant. My wife is straightforward by comparison. She doesn't think in the same dramatic terms of survival and security. She makes unswervingly reasonable assumptions about the future; not that it will always be OK but that, however things turn out, we will find a way to cope. It's a sound point of view, based on precedent.

Why are we built so differently? Maybe it's because my childhood was more chaotic than hers. Or maybe our nervous dispositions are dished out arbitrarily at birth. Either way, I sit there in the car hoping that my daughter's brain is built more like her mum's than her dad's. Finally, she emerges through the gates and walks towards us with an inscrutable half-smile on her face. I make a choking sound. My wife tells me to start the engine. I guess things are going to be OK.

About a month later, both of my kids started new chapters in their education. My son was off to secondary school, my daughter was starting her A levels. I was, as always, more nervous than they were when they set off on the first day. But it all went well; they came back with plenty of tales to tell and big smiles on their faces. 'What the hell was I worrying about?' I asked myself.

Late summer gave way to autumn. The clocks changed and the nights got cold. The novelty of new schools faded and the adrenaline started to run dry. Where once there was optimism and excitement, now there was anxiety, stress and tears. Starting a new school can be brutal. Especially for the parents. They say you're only ever as happy as your unhappiest child. It's true that no matter how well things are going in your personal affairs, it's hard to take pleasure from life when you know one of your offspring is experiencing some sort of pain.

The annoying thing is, it's rarely possible to fix your kids' emotional issues. You can love them, support them and try to understand but you can't ever do what you'd really like to, which is climb inside their mind and manage their thoughts and feelings. Admittedly, it's an unhealthy desire but, deep down, it's what parents crave. We can't handle something that has such a huge impact on our own mood being so far beyond our control. When things are going badly in my own life, I at least have the option of taking a nap or eating a Snickers (the two fail-safe mood improvers that have got me through even the toughest of times).

But if you witness your kid going to school stressed, coming home upset, wondering if things will ever get better, you feel like you're watching from inside a glass box that prevents you from reaching out and touching them. I talk, of course. I talk and talk and talk in the hope it will make things better. The truth is, my talk often seems to make things worse. Stories about my own struggles at school, how I overcame them, what techniques served me well: even as this bollocks spills from my mouth I can hear how boring, irrelevant and archaic it sounds. Like Grampa Simpson trying to explain the olden times to Bart and Lisa.

Here's the quote that sums it up: 'Making the decision to have a child – it is momentous. It is to decide forever to have your heart go walking around outside your body.' Teacher and author Elizabeth Stone wrote that. It's painful to even look at. At the same time, it's reassuring to know that you're not alone and you're not a complete neurotic. You're just a parent and your feelings about your kids cannot be controlled. When it comes to worrying about your children, reason and rationale often take a hike. It's horrible.

I lean on my mum a great deal at times like this. She raised four boys on her own. All of us were troubled and our living circumstances weren't easy. My mum worked full-time and was always exhausted. She wasn't around every minute of the day like I am for my kids. Nevertheless, she always made us feel loved and safe. And, however tough things got, she never showed us anything but total, unswerving confidence. She often lost her shit over her own stuff: her finances, her work, her love life, etc. But when we brought our own problems home she was like Winston Churchill in the thick of World War Two: delivering the most incredibly exhilarating and uplifting speeches that would have me walking out of the front door feeling ten feet tall. It didn't matter if I was crap at football, had fallen out with my mates, had no money in my pocket and couldn't get a girlfriend: my mum could make me feel like a genius, a saint and a rock star all rolled into one.

Yes, she was my mum so I suppose I would expect her to say nice things about me. But she was also a mate. Maybe it was because we all lived squished together in a raucous and ramshackle house. She was just like one of the lads. Funny, noisy, sweary and keen on a Friday night fag with her large Martini Bianco; she wasn't like other mums. We had an extra-special respect for her, I guess.

I'm trying my best to be the same sort of pal to my kids through their times of need. When they doubt themselves, I'll keep my worries to myself and show them the sort of belief my mum always showed in me.

Chapter 15

Stop Shitting Yourself
About Shitting Yourself

So, this is the end of the book – and what have we learned? Quite possibly, fuck all.

I imagine some of you are thinking, *So rest is nice and hard work is a drag? Thanks for the insight, dickhead. Did someone actually pay you to write this?*

My answer is, 'Yes, someone did pay me – but don't worry, it wasn't very much.'

Also, sure, some of this stuff might seem bleeding obvious. But just because we know this stuff it doesn't mean we have the balls to live by it. I have done a lot to take my foot off the pedal over the past decade and the benefits have been numerous. The wheels don't come off the moment you slow down. In fact, life gets better. Not in spite of you slowing down but because of it.

For most of my life, when people asked me how I was, my default answer was 'Good ... busy'. It's a phrase that defines our generation: the presupposed connection between busyness and feeling good. It is stupid. It is grounded in fear of judgement. I have come to understand that busyness and feeling good are not necessarily intertwined – very often, they are at odds with each other. So now, when people ask me how I am doing, I answer, 'Great. I've not really had too much on lately. Thanks for asking.' And, almost always, it's the truth.

We often take life too seriously, getting ourselves worked up about nonsense that doesn't really make a difference and, along the way, we fail to notice all the wonderful things about being alive (like cats and crosswords and unexpected encounters with parrots). Blokes in particular can fall for the idea that they must push themselves towards exceptionalism constantly or they are wasting their lives.

It took me almost five decades to work this out. We are all flung into this world with no training in how to navigate our way. From our first day, we are trying to survive in a chaotic and brutal universe. We must first work out how to not die (as babies we just scream non-stop to elicit nourishment and shelter, then later we take out mortgages and utilise Deliveroo). Next, we have to negotiate with our inner life: the thoughts and feelings that we never asked for but which plague us daily. Worry, fear, pain and panic are always simmering beneath the surface. We stop listening to our own needs and compromise ourselves in order to fit in with others, in the belief that their acceptance will make us safer.

At school, when the exhausting grind of learning, rule-following, social mechanics, hormonal turmoil and undignified PE lessons sometimes land you with perfectly legitimate feelings of sadness and pain, the teachers prescribe 'resilience'. Which is their way of saying, 'Suck it up. We all have to go through this. Stop moaning and get on with it.' So you do.

It continues into adulthood: relationships, identity, ambition, failure, frustration, money, career, health, fitness, booze, drugs and all the other shit you have to work your way through each and every day. We are all winging this shit. Sometimes it can be beautiful. But often it is fucking ugly. And society tells us the same thing our teachers did: be resilient. Suck it up. We all have to go through this. You haven't got it any tougher than anyone else.

And maybe you haven't. But so what?

Parents will often give their kids a speech that starts with: 'Back in my day . . .' It is designed to make the parent feel strong and heroic, a defier of seemingly insurmountable odds, and the child feel weak, inadequate and entitled. The parent will think they are helping by explaining to their child that the only way of surviving this unforgiving world is to bottle up your pain and ignore your feelings. In your twenties and thirties you will often hear older colleagues and bosses give you similar speeches.

I have been on both ends of this messaging in various stages of my life. I have been told by my elders that I must toughen up and knuckle down, and I have given similarly self-aggrandising speeches to my kids and junior work colleagues. It's all bollocks.

You should not feel duty-bound to eat shit in any part of your life. Partly because – spoiler alert – it doesn't always get the results you have been promised. You will not always pass your exams, become a stronger person, climb the career ladder and achieve greatness just because you've suffered in silence while working yourself to the bone. That said, hard work can pay off. Hard work can be a reward in itself. But working hard does not need to define you. Before you start flogging yourself to death, ask yourself why you are doing it. If you are in pursuit of some grand passion then crack on – it is probably worth it. But often we are grafting towards something that we don't really want anyway. If this book is about anything, it's about trying to identify the stuff that really matters to you and the stuff that you have attached value to by mistake, because your peers, society, convention, pop culture or marketing and social media have fed it to you.

The rhythms of modern life just aren't conducive to rest, balance, recovery and comfort. We put ourselves under so much pressure to perform, succeed, compete and progress. More often than not we end up frustrated by the process. Often, we end up disappointed. Always, we end up exhausted. The single biggest improvement in my life over the past ten years has been introducing rest as an essential part of my every day, not just a little bonus that I might find time to squeeze in once in a while. That means not only actual physical rest, whereby I schedule periods of sitting with my feet up in front of the box or going to bed for a half-hour kip in the middle of the day, but also mental rest. I've tried meditation and it never really 'took'. So I switch my mind off in other ways: long walks, gentle runs, video games, listening to whole albums from beginning to end while I sip a cup of tea. Sometimes I make myself drift off to sleep by imagining football matches involving fictional teams. You might think this is odd or pathetic for a forty-nine-year-old man. But the Navy SEALs have a method of getting to sleep quickly while they are on missions called 'box breathing'. Trust me, it takes longer and is much more boring. So I make up football teams in my head instead and am usually out like a light after five minutes.

I'd tried and failed to give up drinking for years before I finally managed to stick with it. The big breakthrough was in my thinking. I had always imagined that being sober represented a sacrifice. I thought only about the things I would have to live without: the buzz, the easy relief, the rewards, the excitement, the spontaneity. I thought that sobriety would require cast-iron willpower – like a monk who resists all bodily pleasures in the service of God. No wonder I never quite managed to quit when I saw things that way. I had painted a mental picture of a completely joyless life of yearning and scarcity. But once I started to visualise a more positive version of my sober self, in which I would gain clarity, energy, self-respect, better health and the trust and admiration of my loved ones, it was no longer a difficult proposition. I had a picture in my mind of a bloke who was capable, self-assured, confident and happy. How you see yourself is so important to what you become. There's a lot of cranky talk about manifesting these days. A lot of it is a load of old cobblers: you cannot think your grandest fantasies into existence. But if you develop a positive vision of the person you want to be then becoming that person is a lot easier.

As it was with booze and drugs, so it has become with rest. When I was younger, I was so hungry for approval, so desperate for admiration, so scared of failure that I never stopped worrying, working or getting wasted. It felt like I was being chased down by wolves and if I stopped trying to outrun them for one moment they would savagely rip me limb from limb. I never pressed pause on my life. I had some success and achieved a few things that I was proud of. But the price I paid was being locked in a cycle of burnout, sickness and volatile mental health.

Sobriety, then lockdown, pushed me into a different life where rest was integral to everything. Again, I had to change my thinking to make it work. For many years I had regarded people who prioritised rest as lazy. My vision of a slower life was based on stoner characters from movies (see Brad Pitt in *True Romance*, Bridget Fonda in *Jackie Brown* or any of the Cheech and Chong movies for reference). I didn't want to be a loser who sat in front of daytime TV eating endless bowls of cereal all the time.

I had experienced that suffocating sort of inertia in my childhood and adolescence and was terrified of ever going back there. But once I started to regard rest as something as nourishing and positive as exercise or eating healthily, everything fell into place. I visualised myself not as a useless layabout but a stronger, fitter, happier and more measured person who was better able to handle the shit life threw at him. I realised that having the confidence to slow down in a world that insists on relentless grind makes you a stronger person, not a weaker one.

But it wasn't just practical, it was a bit political too. I was fed up of hearing morons fetishise hard work for the sake of hard work. I was well aware that many people who grafted all their lives were not necessarily rewarded with riches and happiness. But I also understood that success was unlikely to come my way without a bit of hard work once in a while. So I figured the most important thing in life was to choose exactly what I thought worth working for. I decided that I wanted to maximise the time I could spend having fun with the people I loved. I tried to develop a life that allowed me to work just hard enough to facilitate that.

There are two other things that have helped me achieve my simple goals. First, I stopped giving a shit about what other people thought. Life is short; what is the point of letting anyone shape the way you live it? I am no longer trying to impress anyone (apart from sometimes my kids) and I don't waste time and energy wondering what people think of me. Second, I do just enough healthy stuff to keep me happy, relaxed and ticking over. I'm not trying to be Superman or compete with anyone. I just want to have the energy to enjoy life. I really like this version of myself. Others might find it boring or weird and perhaps they are right. But I am happy and stable. I can regulate my emotions and reflect on my own behaviour better than ever.

Life continues to throw shit at us until the day we die. No work, planning or worrying is ever going to change that. But if we look after ourselves a bit, step back from the mayhem, stop feeling guilty about our own feelings and just calm the fuck down, life feels much less scary. Anxiety is a normal human state. Don't beat yourself up about it too much. But when the fear visits you in the dead of night or on the bus or in the middle of a tedious meeting in the office, just try to let it drift past. Acknowledge it is there, understand the way it makes you feel and have faith in the fact that it will eventually fuck off. It's a lot easier to stop shitting yourself when you eventually learn to just stop shitting yourself.

Acknowledgements

Thanks to everyone who helped this book come about: Matthew Hamilton for his support over the years and Andreas Campomar at Constable for his continued belief. Holly Blood for the excellent editorial advice, enthusiasm, encouragement, professionalism and kindness. It is a privilege to work with you. Also, the brilliant team at Little, Brown: Lucian Randall for the copy edit, David Bamford for the diligent read and extremely helpful suggestions, Meg Shepherd for a great cover and John Fairweather for handling production. Also, thanks Narjas Zatat for running the publicity campaign.

Thanks also to Diane Banks, Matt Cole, Elizabeth Counsell, Martin Jensen and James Bates at Northbank Talent for all the help over the past couple of years.

Also, huge thanks to Paul McNamee at the *Big Issue* for being a brilliant editor for so many years. You have given me the freedom and encouragement to develop many of the ideas that ended up in this book. In fact, some bits of this book originally appeared in my *Big Issue* column and are reproduced here with Paul's kind permission.

Elsewhere in my (so-called) work life: thanks to my podcast partner Andy Dawson for the laughs and the support. Working with you on *Top Flight Time Machine* has helped me to develop a less serious, more enjoyable approach to life. Cheers.

Huge thanks to Jonathan Raggett and his team at Old Government House in Guernsey for giving me the space and time I needed to break the back of this book in early 2024.

I've written a lot about the ups and downs of my life in this book. The one consistent positive since the moment I met her has been my wife, Anna. I've no idea what life would have been like without you. Thanks for being supportive, encouraging, smart, kind, funny and consistently the best thing in my life. To my daughter Coco, I am so proud of you. You're clever, funny, kind, sensitive in all the best ways and more emotionally intelligent than I will ever be. You're also great company and make every day better. To my son, Lenny, we've had so much fun together over the years and will continue to do so for many more. You are clever, kind, funny, brave and compassionate. I love spending time with you and I learn something new from you every day.

Acknowledgements

This book is dedicated to my mum, Bren. Thanks for raising me with love, kindness, intelligence and humour. You're a hero and a legend. I'm not perfect but all the good bits in me I got from you.